MODERN

COLOUR THERAPY

SUE LILLY

Published in 2001 by Caxton Editions
20 Bloomsbury Street
London WC1B 3JH
a member of the Caxton Publishing Group

© 2001 Caxton Publishing Group

Designed and produced for Caxton Editions
by Open Door Limited
Rutland, United Kingdom

Editing: Mary Morton
Coordination and Typesetting: Richard Booth

Title: Colour Therapy
ISBN: 1 84067 296 X

IMPORTANT NOTICE
This book is not intended to be a substitute for medical advice or treatment.
Any person with a condition requiring medical attention should consult a
qualified medical practitioner or suitable therapist.

MODERN
COLOUR THERAPY

SUE LILLY

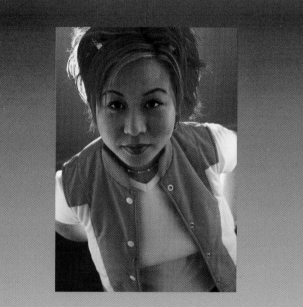

CAXTON EDITIONS

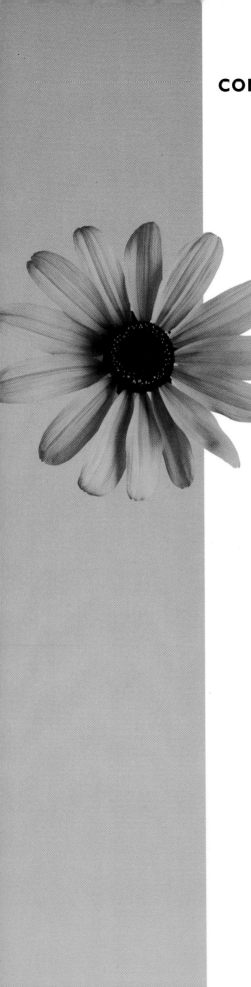

CONTENTS

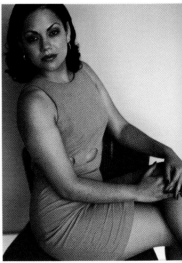

CONTENTS

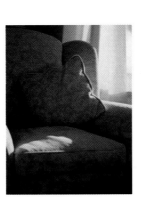
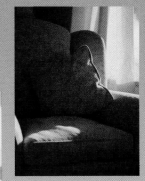

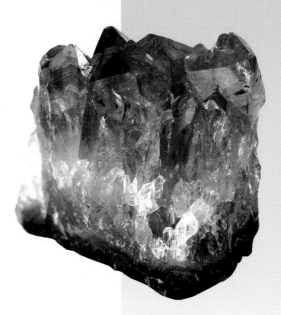

COLOUR – THE HEALING ENERGY ALL AROUND US

Right from when we are very small children we learn to recognise objects by their colour. Bright colours appeal to babies and as we grow we learn to appreciate and distinguish a huge range of very subtle nuances of colour.

Left: right from when we are very small children we learn to recognise objects by their colour.

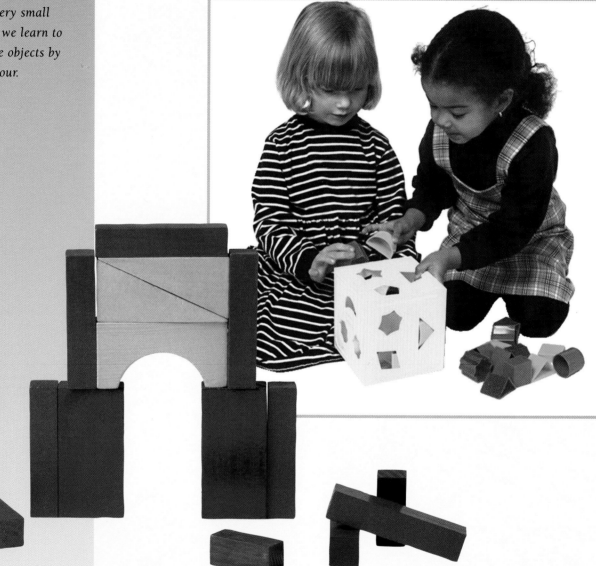

We often find that, amongst the plethora of tones and shades, there are certain colours and combinations that are especially pleasing to us. Likewise, some colours we avoid or ignore. These personal tastes are seldom examined to see how they have arisen or what they might mean. From the perspective of colour therapy and colour healing such personal choices provide a wealth of information about the personality and well-being of the individual.

The sense of sight differs hugely from species to species. Very few animals see the world in the same way as human beings. Colour vision as we would recognise it is available to a small range of animals including the octopus, tortoise and man. So colour vision is in no way universally necessary as a way of perceiving the world. Yet for human beings, colour is very important. This importance can be easily overlooked when we are surrounded by the colour of our daily lives. If, however, we spend any length of time in an environment where there is no colour variation, there grows a sense of the absence of something. This unsettling feeling may remain until we return to surroundings with varied colours.

Colour is emotional food for humans. It "colours" our life, our language, our moods and our thoughts. Colour does this not just through association (i.e. white has a cooling effect, not just because it reminds us of snow), but because it has a real energy that, like heat or sound, affects us at a physical, cellular level. In a way colour is just our method of detecting and recognising the energy of light from stars and identifying what that energy is doing to the objects it is absorbed by or reflected from. As a source of energy, colour is a simple way in which we can regulate and enhance our surroundings as well as improving the way we feel. Colour is a healing energy that can be used by anyone to improve their well-being.

Below: colour vision as we would recognise it is available to a small range of animals including the octopus, tortoise and man.

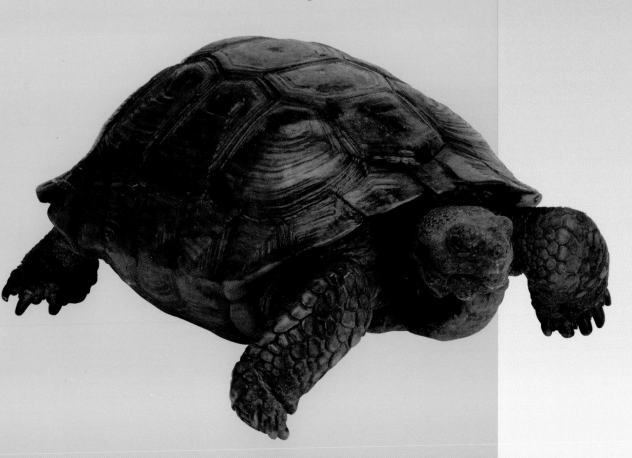

RECOGNISING OUR REACTIONS TO COLOUR

INSTINCTIVE ATTRACTION AND REPULSION: PERSONAL COLOURS

Most of us will recognise that there are some colours with which we feel comfortable and other colours we prefer not to have around us. Such personal choices reflect real differences in our energy makeup and give important clues about the way we choose to act and react in the world around us. Our colour preferences show us clearly where our personal strengths and weaknesses lie. Learning to recognise that colour choices are also a clear reflection of the inner state of an individual can help enormously in choosing which activities and directions are best for our well-being.

Right: personal colour choices reflect real differences in our energy makeup and give important clues about the way we choose to act and react in the world around us.

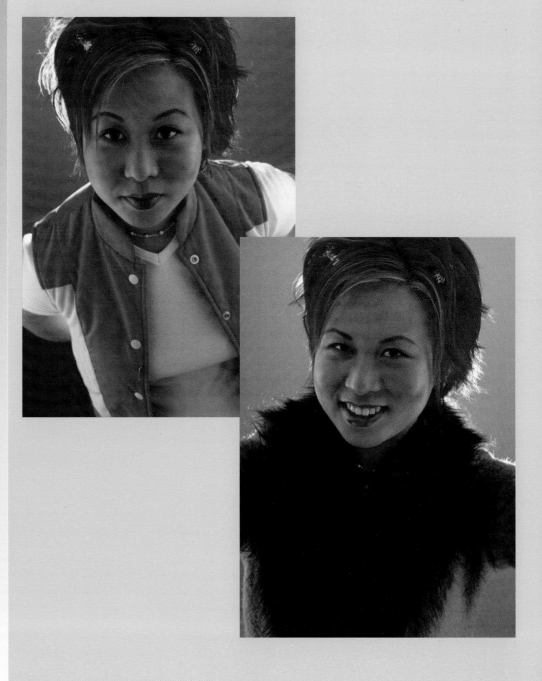

How can a simple preference in colour reveal important facets of our nature?

Left: colour has a real energy and each colour has a different vibration. Each one is a wavelength of light travelling at a different frequency or speed.

The answer lies in understanding that colour has a real energy that affects every aspect of the human being. Each colour has a different vibration – literally. Each colour is a wavelength of light travelling at a different frequency or speed. Red, for example, has a slow, long wavelength that tends to energise chemical reactions. Violet light, on the other hand, has a faster, shorter frequency that tends to pass through matter. Take red to a slightly slower frequency and it becomes infra-red and then microwave energy. Both of these have well known heating effects. Take violet light to a higher frequency and it becomes ultra-violet and then X-rays.

Right: someone who uses a lot of physical energy, who is busy with the practicalities of getting things done, may enjoy the presence of red in their surroundings.

Below: red is a good colour to supply dynamic energy.

Attraction to a colour is thus attraction to a very specific sort of energy. It can show us several different possibilities about ourselves. A favourite colour may represent a type of energy that reinforces our natural qualities. If colour energy is seen as a sort of subtle food, then the favourite colour supplies those nutrients that can be best worked with. For example, someone who uses a lot of physical energy, who is busy with the practicalities of getting things done, may enjoy the presence of red in their surroundings. This colour will naturally help to feed their type of activity when personal energy reserves begin to wane. On the other hand, someone may choose red in order to supply a type of dynamic energy which they feel they ordinarily lack.

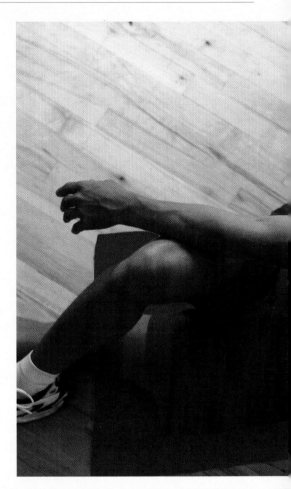

In the first case, the favourite colour reinforces the natural energy of the individual, and in the second case it helps to provide balance by introducing an unfamiliar and underused energy.

A favourite colour that is often used by a person will always reflect the core energy that person needs to maintain their internal equilibrium.

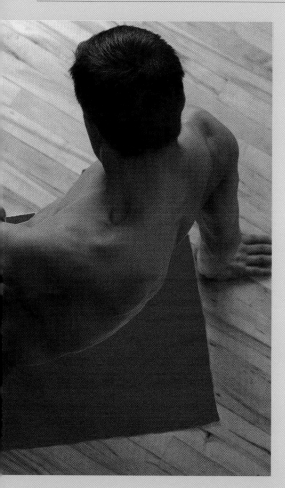

Of all the colours, blue is by far the most frequently chosen as a personal favourite in the western world. Blue has a cool, calming and peaceful energy. Perhaps it is so popular because it is an antidote to the rapid, busy, confusing lifestyles that many of us lead in these days. By way of contrast, red and orange are less popular than green and blue. Where there is too much energy and stress already, these warm colours can aggravate existing imbalances whilst the calming and peaceful energies of the cooler colours can help restore balance.

Our favourite colour can thus reinforce our natural energy makeup or can help as an antidote when we are out of balance.

Below: cool calming and peaceful blue is the colour most often chosen as a personal favourite in the western world.

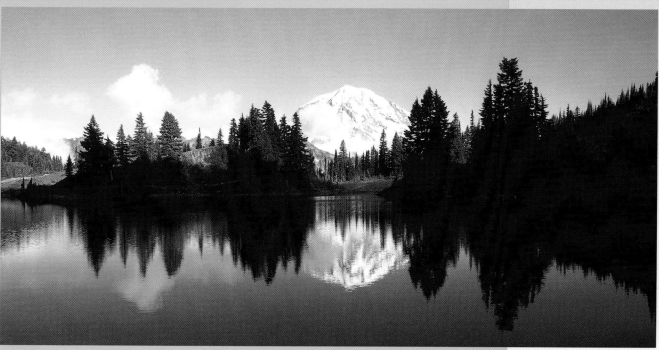

Far right: indigo can create a feeling of isolation, so if you are already feeling isolated another colour is recommended in your surroundings.

Below: a person who is feeling depressed is likely to feel worse if they wear indigo.

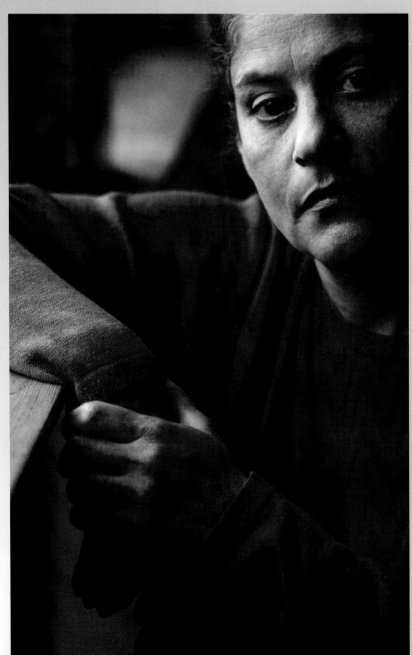

Colours that make us uncomfortable are as important as favourite colours because they clearly show a type of energy that upsets our equilibrium. This can be for several reasons. A colour may be providing too much of a certain vibration. For example, deep indigo has a tendency to create a feeling of isolation or separation from everyday life. A person who is depressed will be likely to feel worse as the indigo energy pushes them

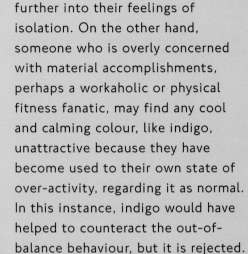

further into their feelings of isolation. On the other hand, someone who is overly concerned with material accomplishments, perhaps a workaholic or physical fitness fanatic, may find any cool and calming colour, like indigo, unattractive because they have become used to their own state of over-activity, regarding it as normal. In this instance, indigo would have helped to counteract the out-of-balance behaviour, but it is rejected.

Favourite colours tell us what energy supports the major aspects of our lives, our basic nature and drive. They do this by keeping us "fed" with that energy, reinforcing it when necessary and supplying extra when we are otherwise lacking.

Colours we reject indicate aspects of our life that we are unwilling to change or deal with, or energies that, in our present state, are felt to be inappropriate to our needs.

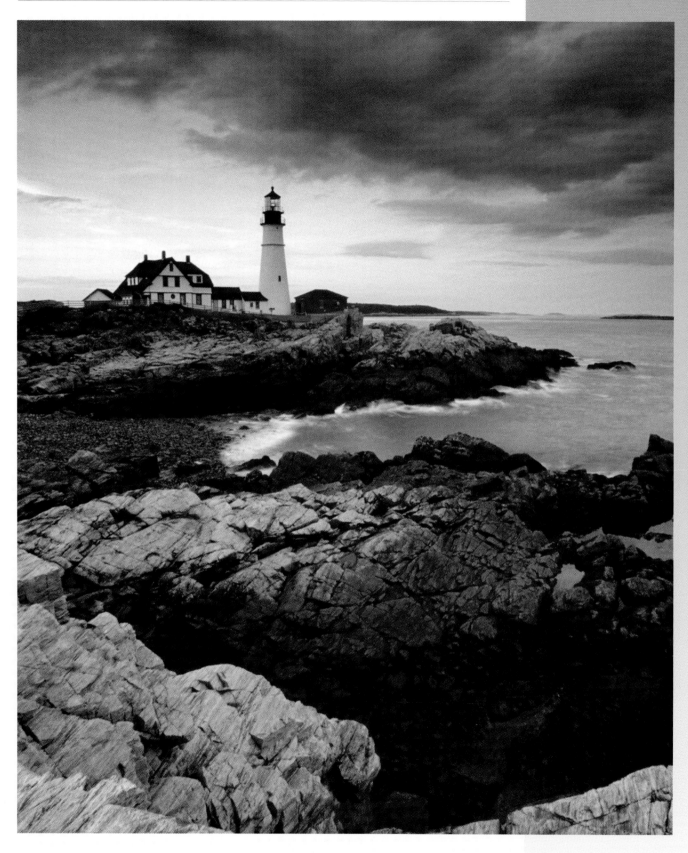

Far right: in western Europe, black is the colour associated with death, and mourning.

Below: a uniform that complies with society's expectations of a person can suppress or deny the expression of personal uniqueness.

REFLECTIVE CHOICE: AWARENESS OF PREFERENCES, INTUITIVE AND CONSCIOUS CHOICE

Because our choice of colour is usually instinctive and immediate, often habitual, it is easy to miss the significance of the colours that we select. A look through the wardrobe will quickly show whether your colour choice is broad or limited. When shopping for clothes do you automatically dismiss certain colours?

Some colours naturally seem to suit a person's skin and hair tone. They look "right" when dressed in a particular colour. However, this is often a fairly superficial use of colour matching that can play down individuality in favour of "corporate flair". A uniform that complies with society's expectations of a person can suppress or deny the expression of personal uniqueness.

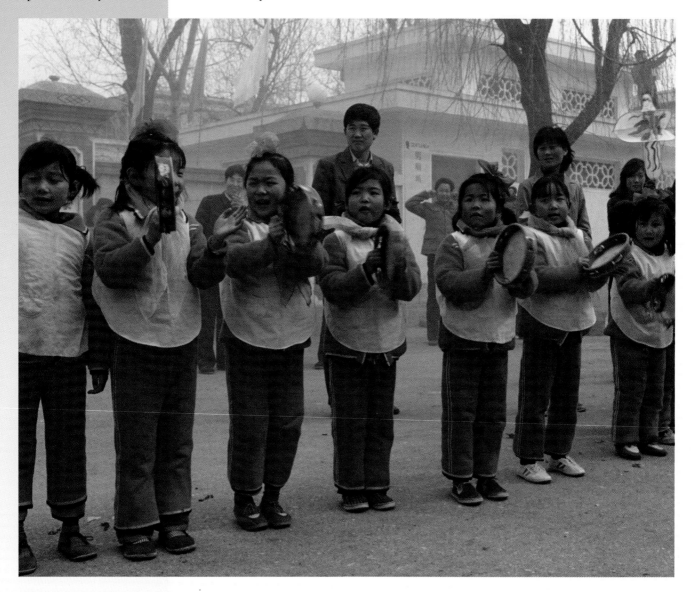

Each society chooses certain colours to represent status and particular important events. In China, white is traditionally the colour associated with death, burial and mourning. In western Europe, black is the colour associated with death. For the last hundred years red has become associated with a very specific belief system, with communism and socialism. Back in the days of the Roman Empire, whole cities became divided into "Reds" and "Blues", each following their own horseracing teams that were sponsored by different political factions and had distinct ideologies. Street battles often raged for days. Wearing the wrong colour could prove fatal. Sports teams, armies and political parties all use colour as an identifying badge. Belonging to one team, we will often consciously choose not to wear the colour of our opponents' teams.

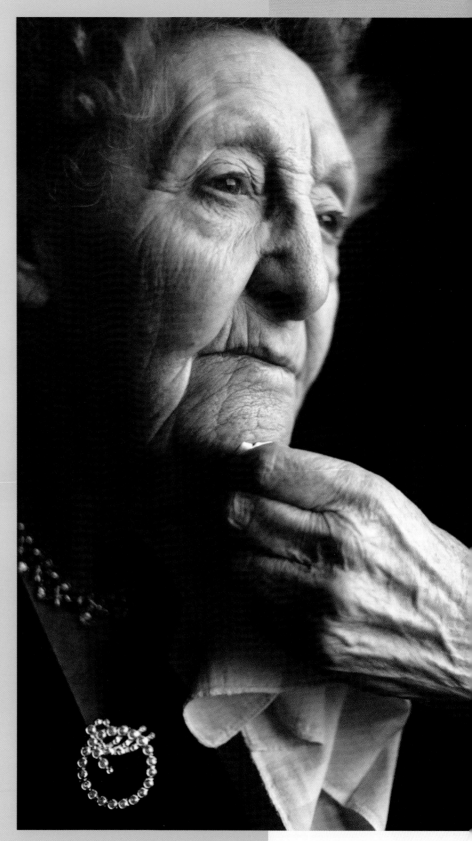

Colour has two languages: a conscious language and an unconscious language; a language of energy and a language of symbol. This is because light and colour interact with the human brain in two different ways. Messages from our eyes travel to the visual cortex of the brain where they are interpreted in terms of sight. This interpretation draws on past experience and things learned from our own culture. It is in this process that colours become associated with specific ideas and beliefs. This colour language usually has some basis in the particular energy characteristics of each colour but in a fairly limited way.

Light that enters the eye also directly energises organs and glands set deep within the middle of the brain. These effects are automatic and outside of conscious control. Here, frequencies of light create changes in how the body functions at profound levels, regardless of what a person might believe a colour symbolises. It is at this level that the language of colour has a universal applicability. It is at this unconscious level that colour can be used to manipulate moods, attract or repulse, create tension or harmony, influence health and well-being.

Below: messages from our eyes, in the form of light and colour, interact with the human brain in two different ways: as a language of energy and a language of symbol.

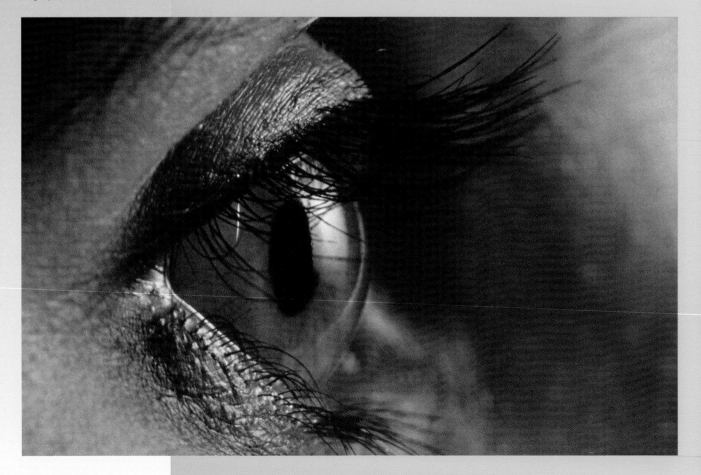

USING COLOUR TO BRING ABOUT CHANGE

Colour has an energy we can all modify and manipulate as we choose. Change the colour and the energy is immediately different. Knowing this, and learning the basic energy effects of colours can definitely bring more control into our lives. With a greater sense of personal power, feelings of confidence and well-being naturally improve. This can be done by making small but effective changes. If your wardrobe is completely navy blue, it is not necessary, or even wise, to throw that out in favour of another colour. It takes time and experimentation to find out how each one of us as an individual reacts to different colours. Certainly if we are able to dress all in one colour for a day, then all in another colour the next day, and so on, it would be an interesting experiment observing how we ourselves and the people around us reacted to the changes in energy. Simple experiments have shown that behaviour patterns alter dramatically as colours change. One test in Canada had a group of people move through and experience a series of rooms, identical except that each was decorated in a single strong colour. Personal preferences were noticed – some people were more comfortable in one coloured room than another. But what was also apparent was the difference in interaction, movement and communication amongst the group as well as their emotional responses. The warm-coloured rooms in red, orange and yellow were energising with lots of chatting and movement, while the cooler green and blue rooms had a quietening, relaxing and calming effect on the way the group behaved.

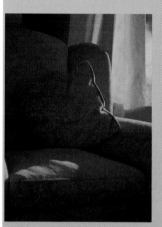

Below: every colour has a different energy. Understanding and learning how to use this by making small changes in our surroundings can have a profound effect and allow us to bring more control into our lives.

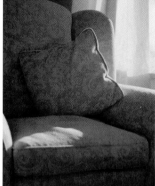

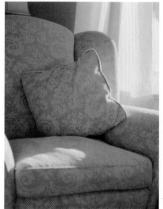

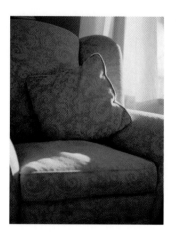

Right: a combination of orange and pink has the ability to ease stress.

Below right: a combination of deep blue and red can give the impression to others of reliability and innovation.

If you have little colour variation in your clothing, or if you are unable to make big changes, then begin with small changes. Using the colour information in this book, introduce colours that will support or improve the activities of your day. If, for example, you need to be seen by others as reliable but innovative, deep blues with a touch of red or orange will give that impression. If you feel unwell or have been upset, a combination of some orange and pink somewhere around you will ease the stress.

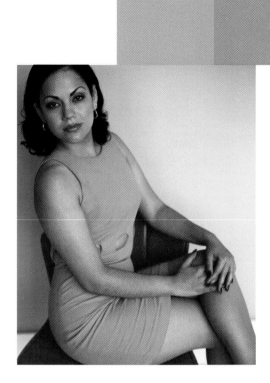

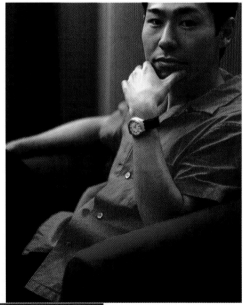

As colours are gradually introduced into your life their energy naturally feeds and stimulates your own state of balance and equilibrium. This means that there will be an increased flexibility and awareness of expanded possibilities in your life. Learning to use a wide range of colour teaches us how to balance the full range of human experience.

There are several ways to select colours for healing and well-being. When we become aware of the important role that colour plays in our lives, it is easy to recognise that we instinctively use particular colours to keep the energies balanced.

It can be difficult to ignore when the desire for a particular coloured item becomes a craving or addiction. For example, one person reported a craving for carrots and oranges that was becoming increasingly overwhelming. On close questioning it was revealed that this had started when they had, several weeks before, experienced a very traumatic event. The body's need to release the shock from the system had resulted in a craving for orange foods. Once this was explained, they were able to take deliberate steps to release the stress, and in a few days the craving had disappeared. The body was instinctively demanding orange as a means to rebalance the body.

In today's world, where we expect communication to be verbal and direct, it is easy to miss or dismiss the language our bodies express through colour.

Below: a shock or upsetting experience can trigger a craving for orange foods.

The choice of colour can also be an intuitive one, made on a daily basis. In answer to the question, "What clothes do I wear today?", or when we are faced with a particular situation, the intuitive choice is the first to come to mind. If the first impulse is ignored, it is easy to find lots of logical reasons why that colour choice should not be made.

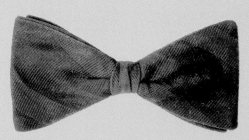

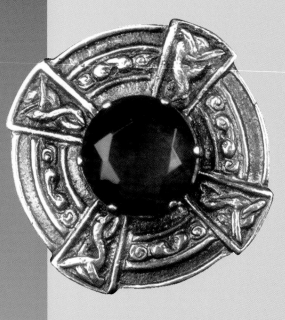

Other ways to select colours centre around the use of coloured items to help focus the current healing needs. The easiest way of making colour selections is through collections of single coloured items. These can be ribbons, buttons, crystals or coloured cards. The collection needs to include all the colours of the rainbow, plus a few extras, like black, white, brown and pink.

Right: the easiest way of making colour selections is through collections of coloured items such as ribbons, buttons, crystals or coloured cards.

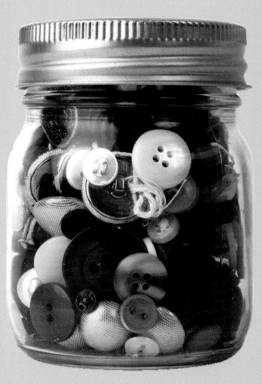

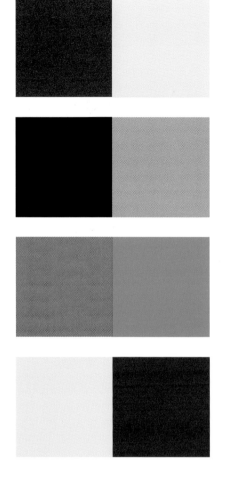

When a specific question is posed, for example, "What colour do I need today for my health and well-being?", an item is chosen. This can be picked out at random. Simply be aware of which colour has drawn your attention the most. The choice of colour that you focus upon can then be used for that day's healing. The colour can be visualised, foods of that colour eaten, or the appropriate clothes, crystals or perfume worn. This exercise can be repeated each day.

Random choice has the advantage over attraction-choice, inasmuch as attraction can be influenced by likes and dislikes. Random choice leaves the decision with the body and its own subtle sensing mechanisms, which are tuned into the energy of colour.

Below: the intuitive choice of colour for each day can be used for healing: visualising, foods of that colour eaten, or the appropriate clothes, crystals or perfume worn.

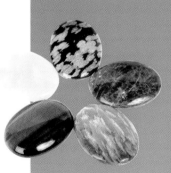

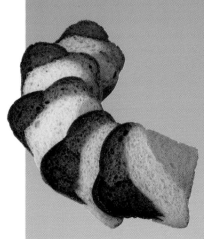

HOW TO USE COLOUR FOR HEALING

Selection can also be made for a more specific healing purpose. For example, the question. "What do I need to help ease this headache?". Your choice here can be very telling. Apart from giving you the healing you seek, a choice of yellow, for example, could indicate an underlying fear or tension. White could indicate a need to detoxify and blue a need for peace and quiet.

More detailed selections can be made when the questions follow a predetermined pattern. An example would be to decide that the:

Next, select the colours and interpret each according to the pre-set structure. The colour listings included in this book will help you to determine methods of using and interpreting the colour choice in practical ways.

First Colour Choice

indicates what is needed for the physical body

Second Colour Choice

represents the colour needed to balance the emotions

Third Colour Choice

for the mental processes

Fourth Colour Choice

for spiritual needs

THE PROJECTION OF COLOUR

Projecting coloured light has always been one of the main techniques used by colour therapists. Very effective healing has been achieved by both shining specific coloured light onto the body and through the eyes. The exact frequency of light and time of exposure is often regarded as crucial. The sequence of coloured lights can also be significant. Specialist equipment and a lot of experience are needed to work safely and effectively in this way. In a few instances it can be very beneficial to shine a colour directly onto the skin. For example, all shades of blue are soothing and can help to reduce the pain of inflammation. Green will have a similar calming effect.

The use of coloured light bulbs or transparent coloured filters is the easiest way to project colour. Even using coloured lampshades can be an effective way of flooding a whole area with a single coloured light.

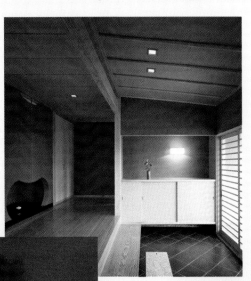

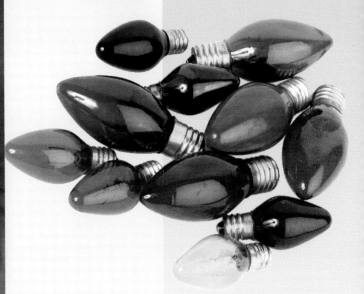

Left: using coloured lampshades can be an effective way of flooding a whole area with a single coloured light.

Below: The use of coloured light bulbs or transparent coloured filters is the easiest way to project colour.

Below left: projecting coloured light onto the body and through the eyes has always been one of the main techniques used by colour therapists.

Below: the power of stained glass windows in churches comes from the dramatic impact of sunlight streaming through bright colours as well as the patterns and imagery.

Coloured sheets of cellophane can be easily taped over windows. Even small coloured areas can be effective – simply gazing through a colour can bring that colour energy into the body. The power of stained glass windows in churches comes from the dramatic impact of sunlight streaming through bright colours as well as the patterns and imagery. Chartres Cathedral is particularly noted for its windows of deep blue glass that create a mysterious, luminous atmosphere of peace and devotion for the worshippers who enter the darkened interior.

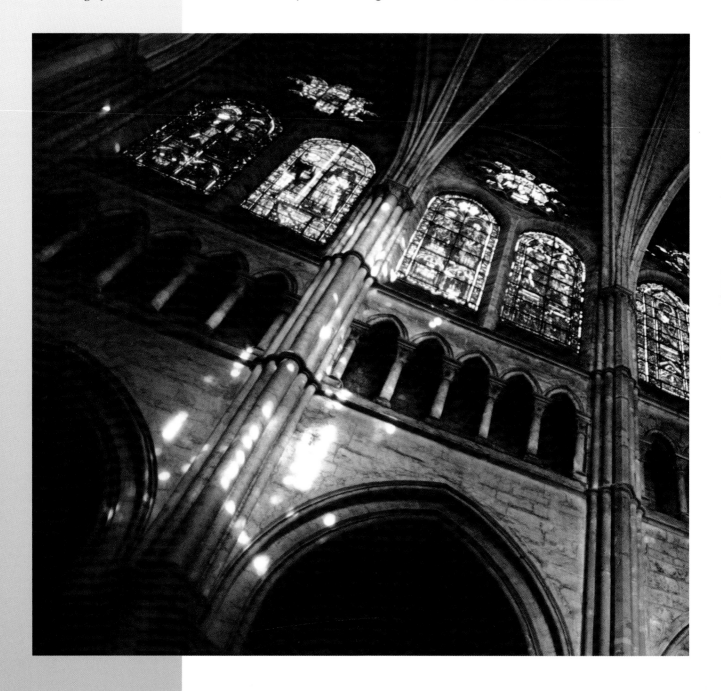

Theatres, too, create changes of atmosphere by placing coloured filters over the spotlights directed onto the stage. These filters, called theatrical gels, are made from sheets of heat-resistant cellulose with very exact colour wavelengths, so they can be combined together to give any desired effect. Specialist theatrical suppliers stock these gels and, although not cheap, they have a jewel-like clarity and transparency perfect for colour healing work. Large sheets can be cut with scissors into manageable sizes and shapes.

Stained glass window effects can be created with these gels and opaque adhesive tape. In this way different tones of the same colour or related colours can be put together to make a dynamic pattern. If it isn't possible to cover a whole window in this way, use a sheet of black paper or thin card to surround the coloured gel. This will also ensure that the room receives a single frequency vibration of light producing a clearer, more dramatic effect on those within.

Above: coloured filters can be used for changing light effects and are perfect for colour healing work.

A slide projector is another useful way to project the vibrancy of coloured light. Theatrical gels can again be used to make single coloured slides. If this is not practical, taking photographs of clear blue skies, other naturally strong coloured objects and weather conditions can work almost as well. The projected colours are bright and vibrant without being damaging to the eyes.

Walking along streets at night, it is often possible to see the wildly flickering colours of television sets in darkened rooms. From outside the colours seem strong and clear, though for the watcher the image usually holds the attention more than the colour it projects into the room. What effect on the human energy system will such strong projections of rapidly changing colour have, even for an hour or so of continuous watching?

VISUALISATION

Visualisation, the ability to think in images, is a natural process of the mind. If you can read and understand these words, you are automatically using visualisation skills. Because visualisation combines understanding with our memories of sense experiences, it re-creates the outer reality of the world inside the mind, free of the limits of time and space. This has a powerful, stimulating effect on the deep areas of the brain that are closely connected with the autonomic systems of the body like the hormones and nervous system. Thinking of a colour stimulates the body in an equivalent way to seeing it with the eyes, so using colour visualisation is an effective method for colour healing.

Although it is a natural skill, visualisation improves with practice. Initially the mind can wander and confidence can waver. It is important to remember that not everyone has the same way of thinking. Some have a strong visual mind, others will have a more auditory (hearing) or kinesthetic (feeling) way of thinking. If you do not habitually think in strong visual images visualisation will tend not to be as clear as watching television! However, with practice sharpness, clarity and depth of colour does dramatically improve.

Below: visualisation is a natuaral skill which can improve with practice: thinking of a colour stimulates the body in an equivalent way to seeing it with the eyes.

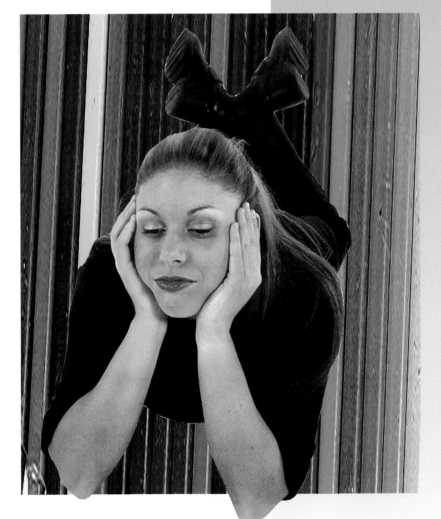

Below: if you are not used to visualisation, at first it is sometimes easier to visualise an object of the desired colour rather than an abstract field of colour.

At first it is sometimes easier to visualise an object of the desired colour rather than an abstract field of colour – a red poppy, a pink rose, a lemon, an orange and so on. This allows the mind to select a real, solid memory to work with. A useful exercise is to quickly run through the colours of the spectrum in your mind from red to violet. It is quite usual for some colours to be seen a lot more clearly than others. Colours that are most difficult to visualise suggest that there is greater need for them at that time. A variation of this simple visualisation can be an interesting assessment of the chakra system.

Simply visualise red light at the base chakra, orange at the sacral, yellow at the solar plexus, then green at the heart followed by a light blue at the throat, a deep midnight indigo at the brow and a violet light at the crown.

As you run through this procedure, you will notice differences in the ability to visualise each colour in its place. Some chakras will be easy to see in a deep vibrant colour, while others will be unclear or muddy – or else will seem to need much more of a colour. This gives an indication of the state of your chakra system as a whole. Spend time at regular intervals reinforcing the colour energies of those areas that proved most difficult to visualise. Notice how you feel as the process becomes easier and more balanced.

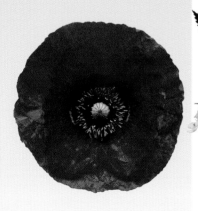

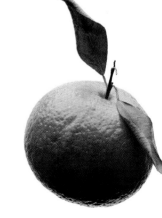

Visualisation can be used to improve the energy of your surroundings by imagining a colour flooding every corner and saturating all objects and people with the colour that seems to be needed. For example, a difficult or argumentative situation would be helped by pink, to calm aggression, and blue, to increase communication. Visualising a bright yellow in yourself and your surroundings will help to increase clarity of mind, decision-making and ability to study.

It may sometimes be useful to begin the visualisation from an object of the desired colour. Simply imagine the colour radiating out from the object until you feel it has filled the space. Another good idea is to begin the visualisation from within your own body, if you can. That way, any internal conflicts will ease, helping you to relax into the most appropriate state of energy.

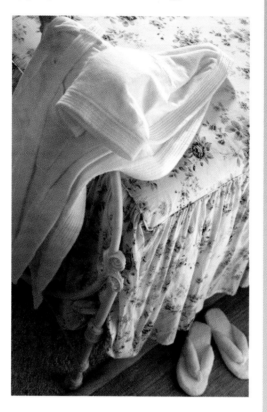

Left: visualising pink will help to calm aggression.

Below: visualising a bright yellow in yourself and your surroundings will help to increase clarity of mind, decision-making and ability to study.

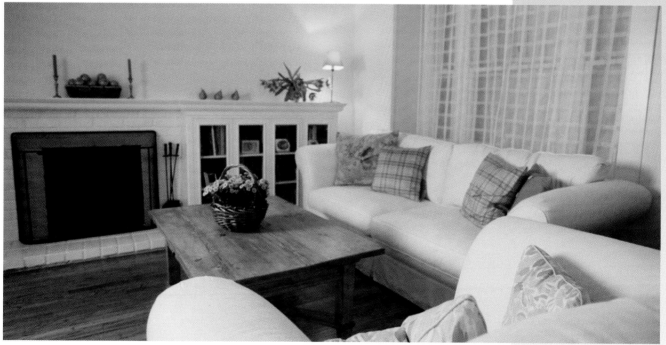

CHAKRAS

Many healers today make use of systems that look at the human body in very different ways from modern medicine. These are drawn from ancient traditions of healing that place more emphasis on spiritual, mental and emotional states. The chakra system derives from Indian traditions and is a very useful method of seeing the body's various energies in a way that makes it ideal for working with colour.

In the chakra system a multitude of physical channels are understood to exist within and around the body. Where these channels of energy meet together, spinning vortices of life-force, called chakras ("wheels") are formed, each one controlling specific functions in the individual body and mind.

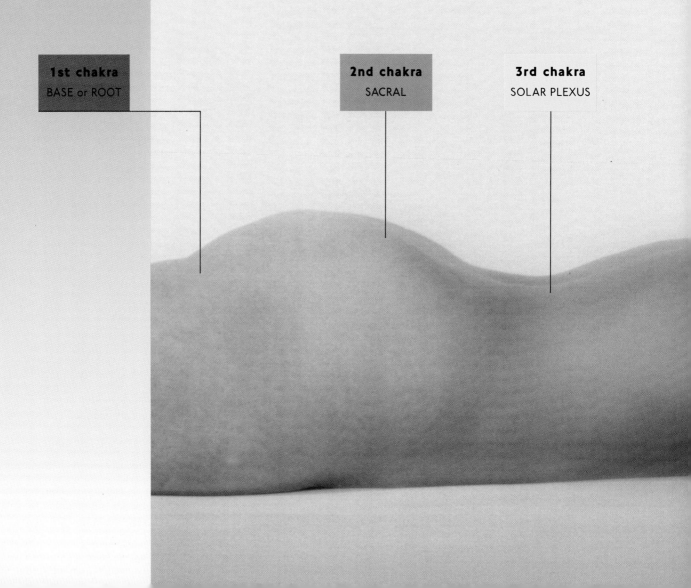

1st chakra
BASE or ROOT

2nd chakra
SACRAL

3rd chakra
SOLAR PLEXUS

Although there are many hundreds of chakras, the most important are seven large centres that lie along the spinal column. It is these chakras that represent the main energies of the body. Their activity and state of balance reflects the behaviour and health of each person. Traditionally, each chakra is associated with particular manifestations of energy represented by complex symbolism. In the West this symbolism has largely been replaced by a simple colour sequence that is easy to remember and work with that, nonetheless, reflects the original designations of each chakra's energy.

The first chakra

This is known as the "base" or "root", is located at the bottom of the spine and is represented by a deep, rich red colour. This chakra is concerned with all issues of life-energy, motivation and survival. It provides the raw energy to all the other systems of the body. It gives solidity to our existence and helps maintain a realistic and practical approach to life. Red also works in the same way, so stimulates the activities of the root chakra. The complementary colour to red, green, quietens the energy of this chakra.

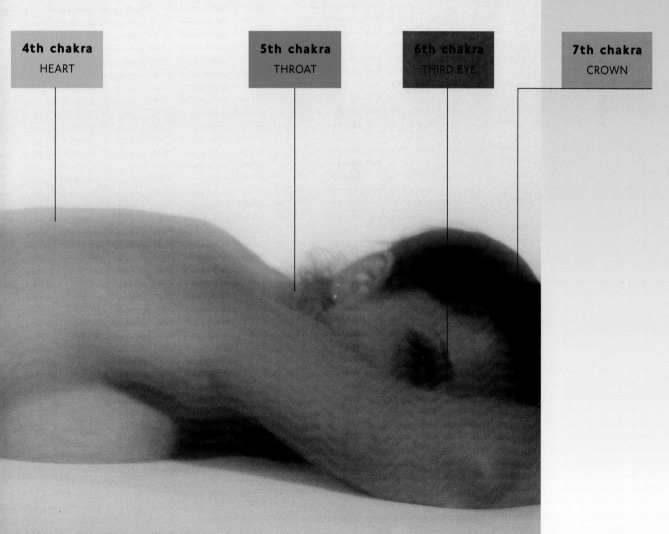

4th chakra
HEART

5th chakra
THROAT

6th chakra
THIRD EYE

7th chakra
CROWN

Below: the sacral chakra has close links with creativity, sexuality and enjoyment.

Between the top of the pelvis and the navel, along the spine, lies the **second or sacral chakra.** This one works with orange energy and with the general energy flow within the body. It has close links with creativity, sexuality and enjoyment. The sacral chakra motivates us to explore the world through our emotions and senses. Blue will quieten the energies of this chakra.

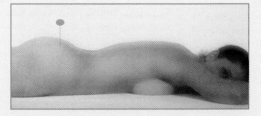

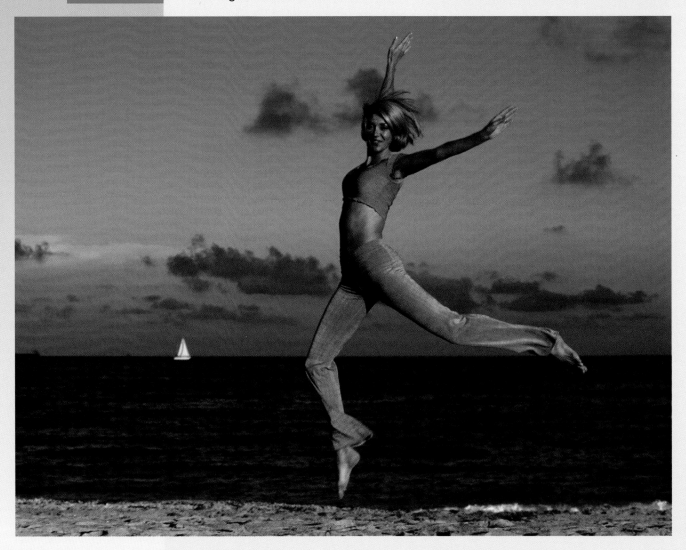

The third chakra

This is located at the solar plexus, just beneath the ribcage. It is linked to yellow and is concerned with organisation at every level of the individual. It provides the ability to discriminate life-supporting from life-damaging energies, brings clarity of thought, maintains personal power and helps to digest information and food. All types of digestive upset, over-sensitivity to the environment, poor immune system and poor memory show disruption at the solar plexus chakra. Yellow will activate this chakra, violet will quieten it.

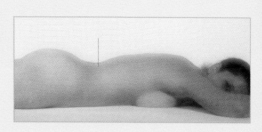

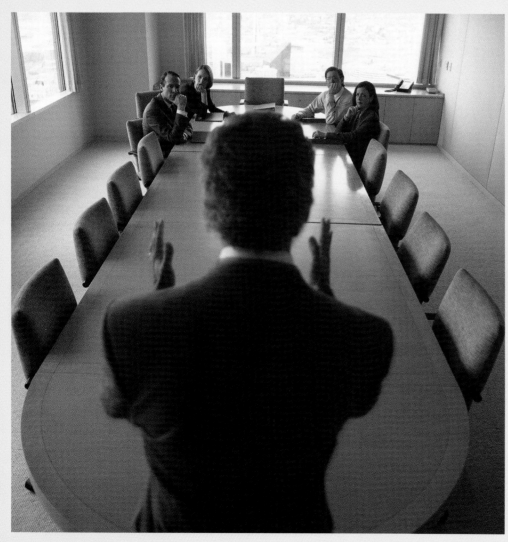

Left: the solar plexus chakra is linked to yellow and is concerned with organisation at every level of the individual.

Below: relationship, understanding and acceptance are all properties of the heart chakra as well as personal direction and growth.

Right: the throat chakra is linked to blue, with a primary function of communication.

The fourth chakra

The heart chakra, is in the centre of the chest. It is linked to green and its function is to bring overall balance to the entire system. Relationship, understanding and acceptance are all properties of this chakra. Personal direction, growth, expansion and a good sense of personal boundaries show a balanced heart chakra. The complementary colour, red, turns the energies of the heart centre away from other people and more towards the self, reflecting the qualities of the root chakra.

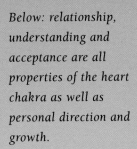

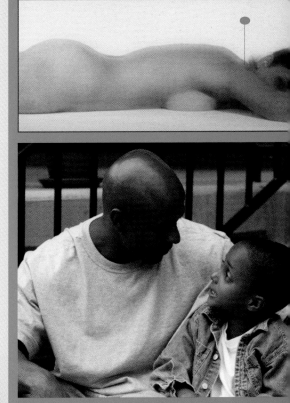

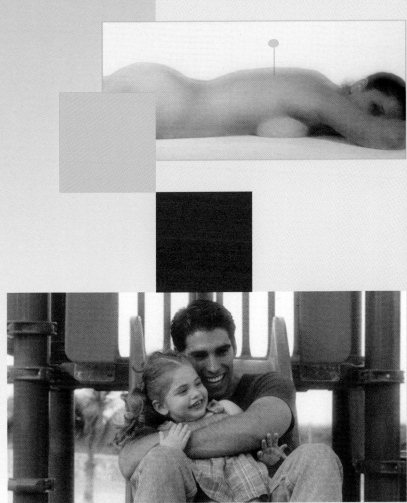

The fifth chakra

This can be found at the base of the throat and is usually referred to as the throat chakra. This centre is linked to blue, with a primary function of communication. Expression of personal thoughts, ideas and emotions and of received information, such as teaching are all covered by this chakra. Like its complementary chakra, the sacral, the throat chakra encourages a flow of energy through the body. Orange energy and the sacral chakra focuses the flow inwards, whereas the natural flow at the throat chakra tends to be outwards. Any difficulty in communication shows a need for blue energy to balance the throat chakra.

The sixth chakra

This is at the centre of the forehead, and is called the brow chakra or, more popularly, the third eye. This corresponds to the colour indigo and is concerned with all processes of understanding and making sense of the world. It helps to process imagery, and creates a context for our perceptions. This chakra also deals with intuition and imagination. When the brow chakra becomes out of balance and drifts into delusion and fantasy, the clarity and organisation of a lemon yellow can help to quieten and integrate its energies.

Below: the brow chakra or the third eye corresponds to the colour indigo and is concerned with all processes of understanding and making sense of the world.

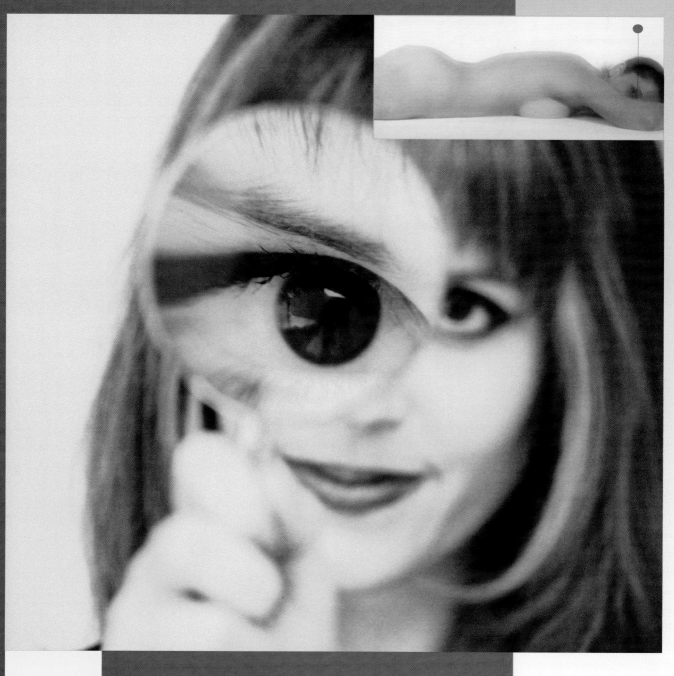

The seventh chakra

This is called the crown chakra, and is located slightly above the top of the head. This chakra equates to the colour violet and with the spectrum as a whole. The crown chakra connects the individual to the rest of the universal energies and is the control centre for the whole chakra system. Its function is to focus consciousness and fine energies into the physical body. The gold colour related to the solar plexus harmonises and balances this chakra and helps with the process of integration that is stimulated by violet.

The chakra system works as an integrated whole. Should one part become unbalanced, the rest will also be affected. As in all colour healing it is wise to remember that all colours are needed for well-being. Individuals will show particular strengths and weaknesses that will favour particular colours and chakras at certain times, but an overall balance needs to be maintained with the whole spectrum of colours.

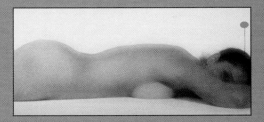

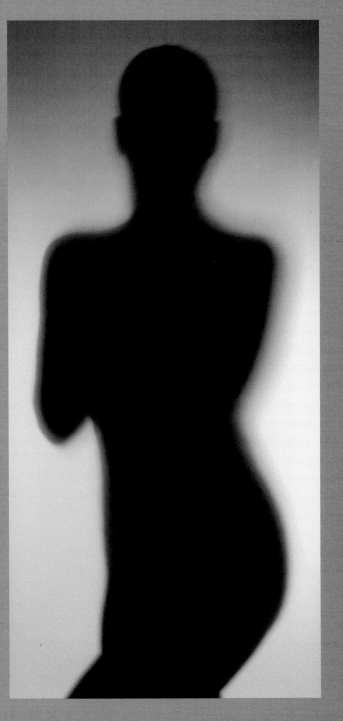

Right: the crown chakra connects the individual to the rest of the universal energies and is the control centre for the whole chakra system.

ENVIRONMENTAL CHANGES, CLOTHES

Whilst coloured light reflects around the whole of a space, colouring everything with that special energy, coloured objects have a more restricted, but still significant, effect on us as they catch our eyes.

Because our energy needs are continually changing, it may be wise to adopt a flexible approach to the colours we choose to live around. Even a favourite colour can become overwhelming and oppressive if it isn't balanced by other colour energies. This is especially pertinent in those rooms and areas in which a lot of time is spent. A balance should be sought where colours complement and support the functions of the room as well as the preferences of the main inhabitants.

Designers use the psychology of colour to create the right feel for a space and can easily alter our perceptions by a change in tone or colour. Light colours will always make a space feel bigger and brighter whilst darker colours will reduce the apparent size of a room and reflect less light from windows. It is usually considered that red is not a good idea in a bedroom as its energy can prevent the body from settling down to sleep. The favoured colours are soft pinks, blues and violets – colours that resonate with rest and quietness. But these guidelines are general and not necessarily the best for every individual.

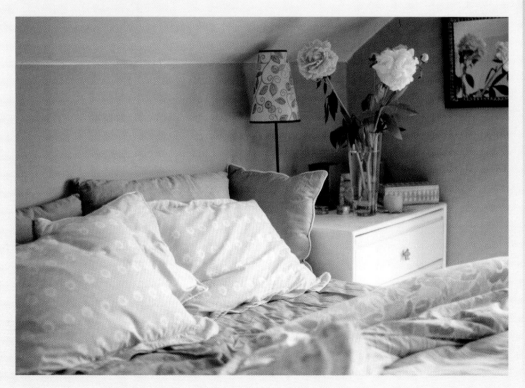

Left: in a bedroom the favoured colours for a peaceful night's sleep are soft pinks, blues and violets – colours that resonate with rest and quietness.

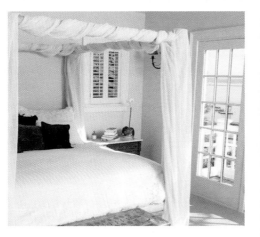

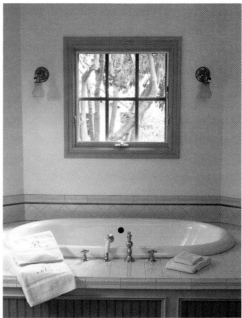

Right: when deciding on colours for decor, consider the main energy needed in each room.

Consider the main energy needed in each room: restful for bedrooms; refreshing in bathrooms; comfortable and cosy for living rooms; elegant in public rooms; clean and bright for kitchen and dining areas. Choosing overall colours with subtle tones and shades allows dramatic statements of colour to be included in furnishings and changed whenever needed to support well-being and health.

In each area of a home consider what aspects could do with improvement or whether your overall health might benefit from the input of certain colour energies. For example, poor appetite can be stimulated in the kitchen or dining area with even a small amount of bright yellow, whilst dullness and confusion in a study or work area will be reduced by careful use of lemon yellow.

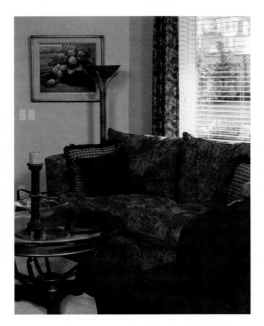

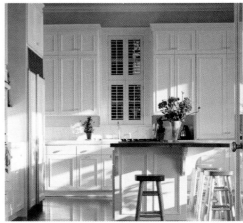

Use of complementary colours creates a dynamic effect that enhances both colours. Used in moderation, this can create a very balanced energy. Complementary colours are:

Black and white
Red and green
Orange and blue
Yellow and violet
Magenta and turquoise.

Clothing can be selected in the same way. Wearing colours that you like will naturally help to support your own individual energy, but when you know you lack a certain type of energy, or where there is a need for a different type of behaviour, add a small amount of the appropriate colour. Even if it is not possible to dress totally in bright pink to bolster your confidence in a threatening situation, a pink scarf, tie, underwear, ribbon, flower – will all contribute to that helpful energy.

As coloured material like clothing is reflecting a certain part of the spectrum of light, whether the item is visible to us or not, our body at some level is able to recognise and make use of that energy when it is needed – even if it is covered by several layers of clothing or shoved deep into a pocket.

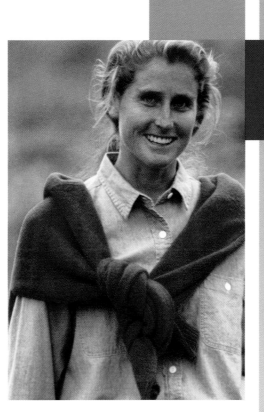

Left: used in moderation, complementary colours can create a very balanced energy.

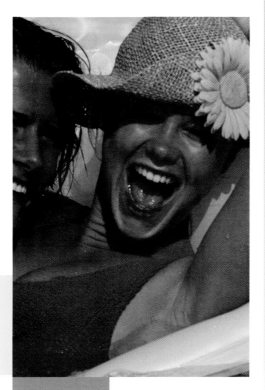

Below left: if it is not possible to dress entirely in the colour you need to boost your energy, a scarf, tie or flower in the appropriate colour will contribute.

Below: the visual effect of the colour of food is an important trigger to the digestive processes (as is the smell). Food that looks appealing is easier to digest.

COLOURED FOODS, COLOURED WATER

The food we eat is a natural way to absorb the colour energies we need. From a nutritional point of view each colour often represents concentrations of particular vitamins and minerals. Add to this the fact that every frequency of colour stimulates different types of chemical activity in the body and it makes sense to take notice of what sorts of food we are drawn to eat.

The visual effect of the colour of food is an important trigger to the digestive processes (as is the smell). Food that looks appealing is easier to digest. Experimentation with harmless dyes has shown that it is difficult to eat even our normal foods if they have unfamiliar colours – particularly blue and black. Food manufacturers try to make food more appealing by strengthening and brightening the natural colouring of foods with additives, whilst supermarkets carefully light their fresh food areas to emphasise the greenness of vegetables, the red of meat, and so on.

One way to emphasise the full range of colour energies in the diet is to consciously choose as wide a range of coloured foods as possible in each meal. In this way the visual stimulus to the digestive processes is strengthened and at the same time colour energy affects the areas of the brain concerned with sight.

Solarised water has been a simple method of using the healing power of colour for at least a hundred years. Pure water in a glass or jug is placed in full sunlight with a coloured filter over it. The effect of sunlight passing through the colour into the water charges the water with the energy pattern of that colour. The water can then be sipped throughout the day, or, if it is needed over several days, stored in a fridge. Mixing this solarised water with about equal amounts of brandy or vodka will preserve it indefinitely. A few drops can then be taken as and when that colour energy is needed. If solarised water is placed in a little hot water, the alcohol will evaporate without effecting the healing properties of the water. Flower essences are made in a similar way except that, instead of a coloured filter being used, flowers of the required kind are floated on top of the water in sunlight for a couple of hours.

The remarkable thing about solarised water is that the taste of each coloured water has a distinct quality even when the water is from an identical source and prepared at the same time. Somehow the coloured light changes the nature of the water in a way the body can recognise, even though it may look no different from water from a tap or bottle.

Solarised water is a vibrational, energetic form of healing and so is effective in very small amounts. Sipping a little on a regular basis, or placing a few drops on a part of the body needing healing can have speedy results.

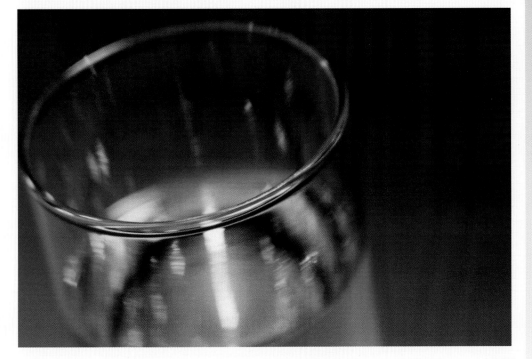

Left: solarised water has been a simple method of using the healing power of colour for at least a hundred years.

Below: clear quartz crystals and a selection of tumbled stones. Crystals have unique physical and energetic properties.

CRYSTALS

Crystals and gemstones have been used for thousands of years both for decoration and healing. Colour that is brilliant and enduring is clearly one of their attractive features. Crystals are simply the most organised and perfectly balanced examples of physical matter in the entire universe. They are created where atoms are able to come together in the most stable of arrangements.

It is this level of stability that gives crystals their unique physical and energetic properties. The three-dimensional pattern of atoms, known as the crystal lattice, is responsible for the geometrical form and colour of each crystal.

The visible colour can come from the inherent colouring of some of a crystal's constituents. For example, minerals containing atoms of sulphur will show a yellow colour, and those with copper atoms will tend to be green. But many types of crystal can appear in a great variety of different colours and this is caused, not by the types of atoms involved, but more by their arrangement in space. This causes the rays of light passing through to become distorted and moved towards a different part of the light spectrum. The most highly prized crystals, used as gemstones, tend to be those that are highly coloured and transparent. Colourful, opaque or translucent crystals that reflect light or allow only some rays into the stone, have mainly been considered less valuable, semi-precious stones.

For the colour healer, all stones, whatever their chemical makeup, geometrical shape or gem quality, can become useful tools that concentrate the energy of colour in a small area, yet can affect a significant space around them. From a practical viewpoint crystals provide strong, permanent colour in a durable form. Energetically, because of their inherent orderliness, crystals can have a more powerful influence than just colour alone would provide. As a general guide, all stones of a colour range will provide different aspects of that colour energy. Thus garnet, ruby and jasper are all commonly red. Garnet, as a deep, clear transparent red, will be profoundly energising, whilst ruby has a softer red colour and tends to be less fiery, offering a more stabilising and sustaining influence. Red jasper, an opaque variety of quartz, on the other hand, brings practical, grounding energy.

Below: red jasper and garnet, both red stones with slightly different energising qualities; garnet, (left) being deeply energising and red jasper, (centre and right) bringing a practical, grounding energy to the wearer.

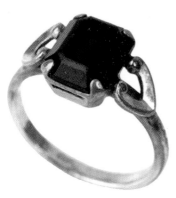
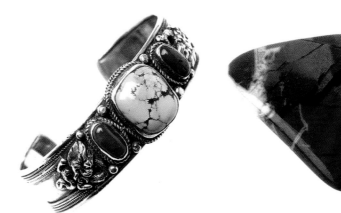

Below: crystal jewellery is an obvious way to bring the most appropriate colours into the personal energy field.

Having a wide range of crystals and semi-precious stones will allow you to select the most appropriate energies for any need. The simplest way to make a collection is with tumbled stones. These are pieces of crystal that have been polished with successively fine grades of abrasive gravel until they become smooth and shiny. The advantage with tumbled stones is that they tend to be relatively inexpensive and are less prone to damage than the delicate edges and points of natural crystal forms.

Crystal jewellery is an obvious way to bring the most appropriate colours into the personal energy field. Necklaces, pendants, earrings and rings can all be found with many different stones and colours. Simply carrying a tumbled stone or two in the pocket will help to introduce that colour vibration into your activity.

Larger, more impressive single pieces, or collections of coloured stones can effectively be placed around a room to bring needed colours into your immediate surroundings.

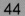

FLOWERS AND ESSENTIAL OILS

Flowers have been used since time immemorial as offerings to others on special occasions. The variety of colour and shape makes them endlessly fascinating. Bringing the beauty and vibrancy of the natural world into a room immediately enlivens the atmosphere. Choosing a bunch of appropriately coloured flowers can bring healing at many other levels as well. For instance, orange and pink together make a healing combination for those recovering from illness, surgery or accidents because they encourage repair to the subtle energies of the body as well as helping to remove toxins, calm emotions and improve self-confidence.

Red roses, traditionally given as a token of love, combine the red petals of passionate energy with the green leaves of a balanced heart and emotions.

The scent of roses, too, evokes the warm, sensuous nature of the flower. Perfumes, scents and incenses, although not coloured themselves, can be useful because of the recognised energy relationships between them and the plants they originated from. Both colour and smell elicit deep, automatic responses within the powerful, unconscious areas of the brain. Scent can, even more than colour, elicit strong memories and emotions. Very

often the qualities of essential oils are categorised by their colour-related actions on the body. Oils and incenses that are heavy, earthy, rich and stimulating can be used for "red" energy. Such oils as patchouli, clove, ylang ylang, black pepper all work in this way. Care should be taken, however, as our preferences for scents are even more individual than our colour choice. One person's stimulating, beautiful, rich, sensuous perfume is another's cloying, nauseous, migraine-inducing smell! Like colour, essential oils have powerful effects on the emotions, so be aware of any changes in mood. Using an oil-burner, with one or two drops of the essential oil in the water, can be the most effective and safe way to utilise their healing ability.

Below: red roses combine the red petals of passionate energy with the green leaves of a balanced heart and emotions.

Below: essential oils made from Sandalwood, ginger and cedar all soothe and balance in an "orange" way.

Essential oils that correspond to the yellow vibration tend to be sharp, pungent and clearing to the mind. Lemon oil, citronella and grapefruit can all be used when we lose our focus, feel tired or need to study.

Right: essential oils that correspond to the yellow vibration tend to be sharp, pungent and clearing to the mind, such as grapefruit.

"Orange" oils are warming, helping the digestive processes and are generally restorative. Essential oil of orange blossom, called neroli, as well as other oils derived from the orange tree – petitgrain and orange – can help to relieve stressful times. Sandalwood, ginger and cedar all soothe and balance in an "orange" way.

The vibration of green energy is found in essential oils that work well with clearing and balancing the body. Pine, eucalyptus and cajeput all help to clear the airways of the lungs and sinuses. Basil, mellisa and bergamot have calming qualities, relaxing the body and lifting the emotions. Many plant oils share blue and green qualities. Thyme, sage, rosemary and peppermint all bring clarity to the mind and help to stabilise body functions. Soothing and sedating oils exhibit characteristics of blue energy. Chamomile, lavender and valerian are all used to promote relaxation and sleep.

Geranium and rose oil complement the use of pink as a gentle way to restore ease and confidence, bringing a warmth and comfort to body and mind.

As in all the many ways of using colour for well-being, the use of fragrance should be subtle and balanced. Intense exposure to the balancing energies of a specific colour or scent can be helpful in small doses, but will quickly become overwhelming without variety. Remember the energies represented by the spectrum of coloured light are all equally valuable and needed in our lives. Don't create a new imbalance by focusing too much on one type of energy at the expense of all the others.

Below: the green energy of basil has a calming quality, relaxing the body and lifting the emotions.

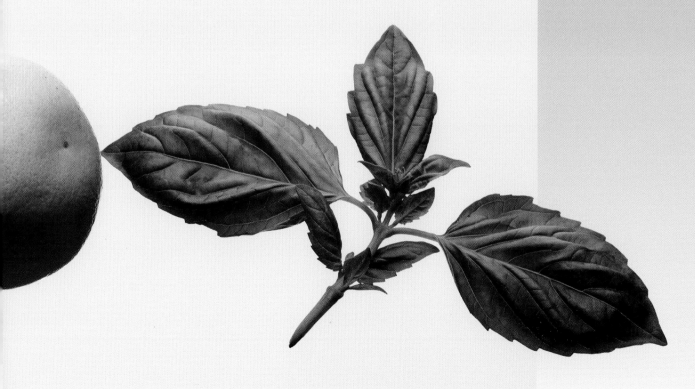

BLACK

Black is not technically a "colour", but the absence of any colour. Instinctive reactions to black suggest an innate response to this absence. For some, black is to be feared, representing emptiness, evil and a void that touches a hidden place deep inside. To others it is a safe, impersonal haven where individuality can be lost.

In the symbol commonly known as Yin-Yang, the balance of the opposites, black and white, is clearly seen. The experience of black automatically gives a glimpse of white because neither can stand in isolation. Without one we cannot clearly identify the other. An extreme attraction or aversion to black can thus be interpreted as an unwillingness to allow any growth, movement or possibility.

Below: the experience of black automatically gives a glimpse of white because neither can stand in isolation.

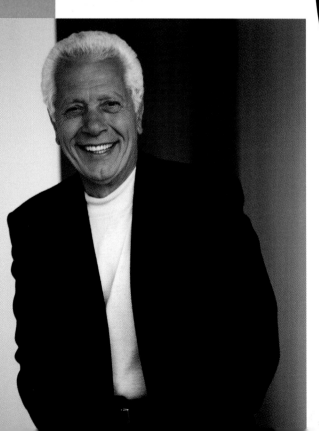

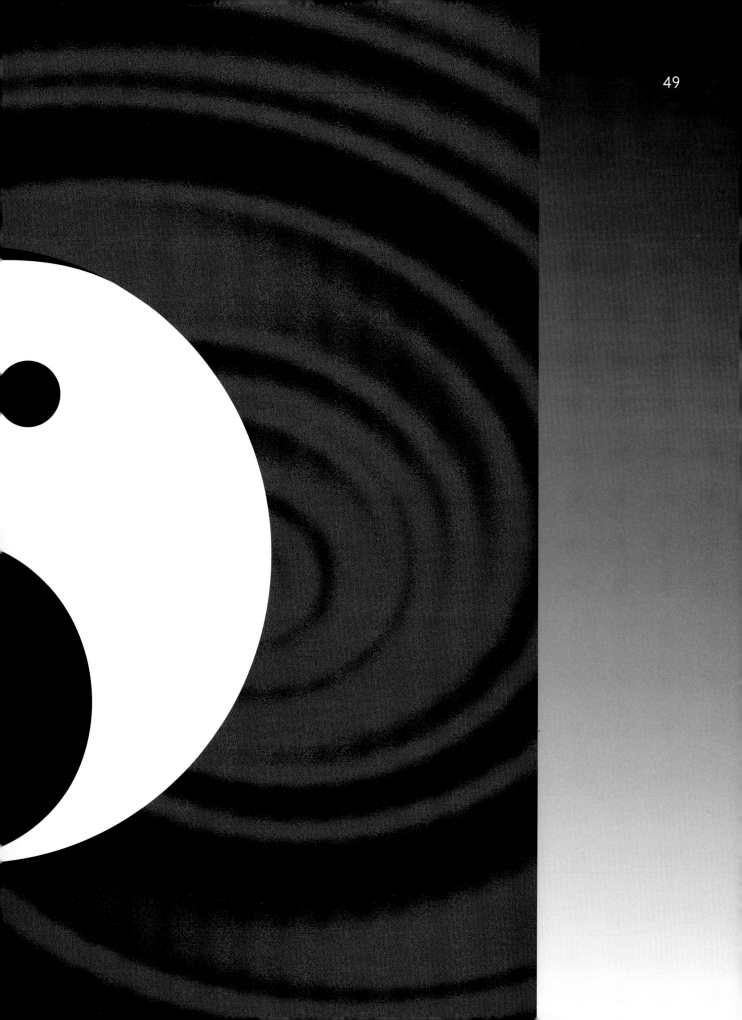

*Right: wearing black
clothes keeps someone
safe from the unwanted
attention of others. This
creation of a protective
shield allows the wearer
to go unnoticed in their
immediate
surroundings.*

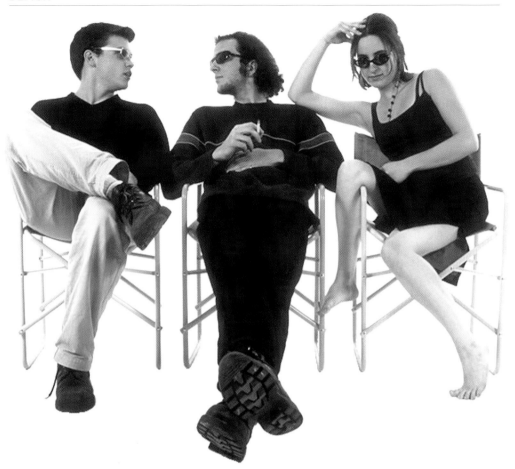

Physically, black creates a holding energy that, depending on the situation, can be a help or a hindrance. It absorbs all forms of energy. Wearing black clothes keeps someone safe from the unwanted attention of others. This creation of a protective shield allows the wearer to go unnoticed in their immediate surroundings. As soon as a splash of colour or decoration is added to black, the anonymity ceases and the black serves to highlight and enhance the individual and their appearance.

Emotionally, black can provide a respite from many strong emotions. By reminding us of the impersonal darkness of night-time and the safety of womb-like places, black can create an energy into which to withdraw. For short periods this can be very healing. Deeply held emotions that have been buried can be brought to the surface to be dealt with. All through our lives, when we fail to fully experience the pain in situations, the unprocessed emotions get locked into our "shadow self". This is sometimes called our "dark side" because we know it holds our collection of painful emotional baggage. Working with black crystals, such as smoky quartz, black tourmaline or with the volcanic glass, obsidian, can help to access the hidden emotions and begin the integration of our shadow self.

Mentally, black can reveal the hidden depths of our mind. This can also be related to the shadow self, to the thoughts that unconsciously direct our lives. When thoughts are allowed to arise and fade without attention paid to them or action taken on them, the mind reflects the potential of black. Many people do not allow themselves enough quiet time to experience this aspect of the mind. When attention is first turned within there can seem to be a barrage of thoughts that some may perceive as to be outside of themselves or as a result of some malefic influence.

Filling our time with activity and constant stimulation effectively cuts us off from the awesome depth and potential of the mind, and denies us access to that part of our shadow self. In this way we do not get chance to discover our hidden skills. Taking time out by ourselves, to become familiar with our own company and our thoughts can ease all this. By sitting quietly with eyes half-closed, allowing thoughts to come and go, paying no attention or giving no encouragement, helps to experience black at a mental level.

Below: black at a mental level allows time out from stimulation and activity and encourages the free flow of thought without encouragement.

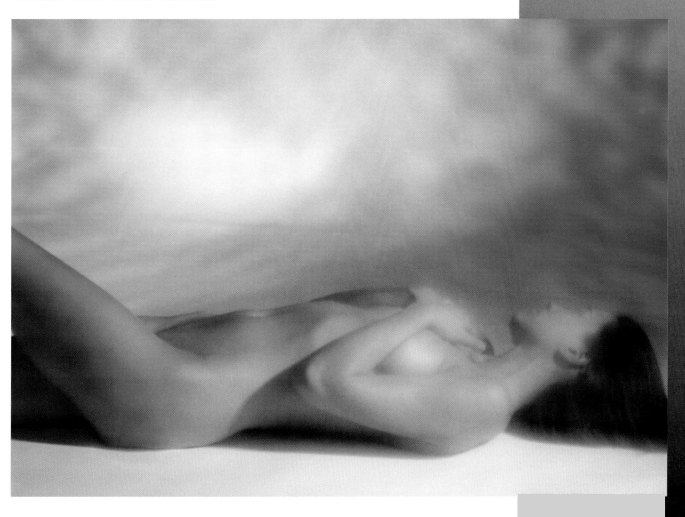

BLACK

Spiritually, black represents the exploration of the depths of the mind. By allowing black to become part of everyday experience, the emptiness of the mind holds no fears. When thoughts do arise, their beauty and the clarity of the perception of those thoughts carries a spark of joy in creativity that is unsurpassed.

SUMMARY:

To balance the black energy in your life:

Spend time alone, practising "being" rather than "doing" or thinking about "doing".

Use black crystals:

smoky quartz, obsidian, black tourmaline

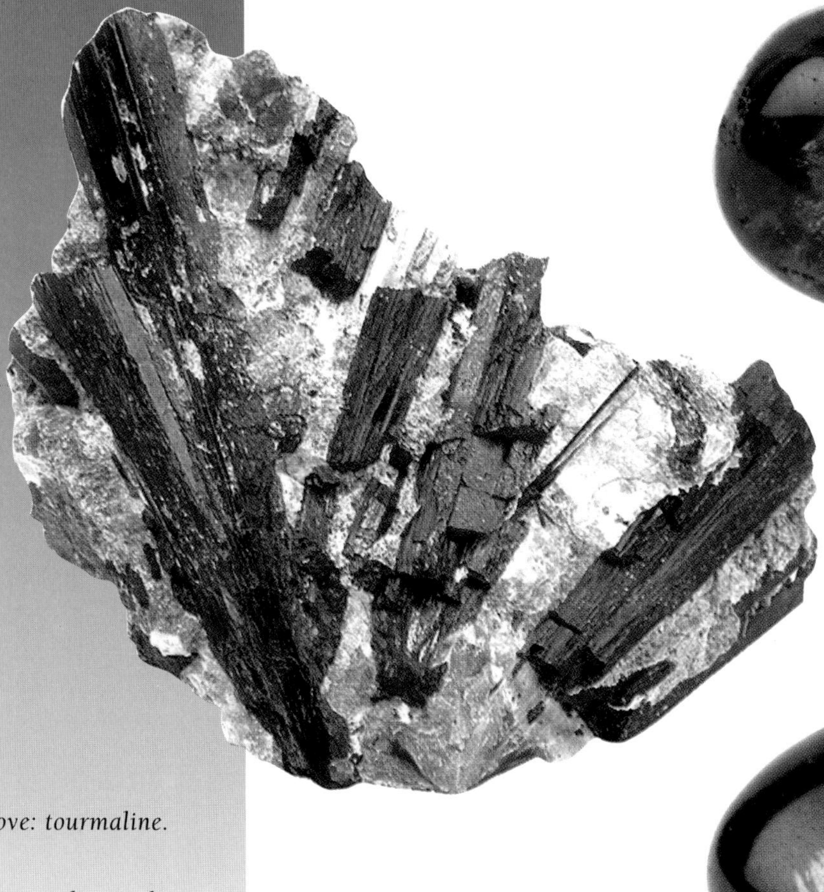

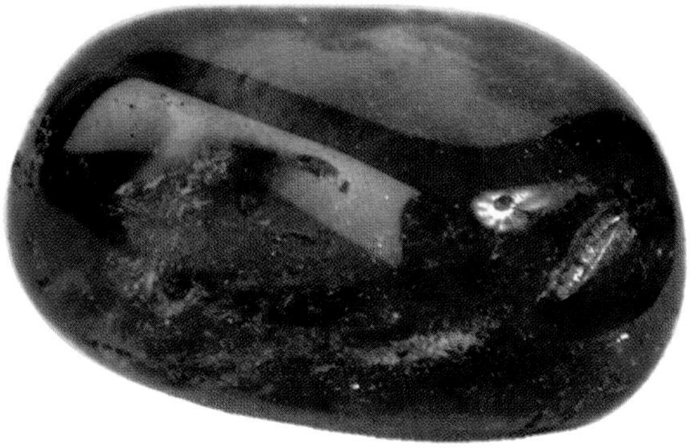

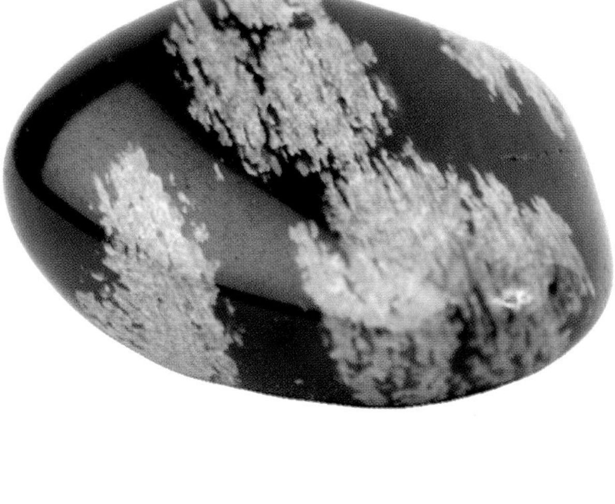

Above: tourmaline.

Above right: smoky quartz.

Right: obsidian.

Red throughout history has connotations with life and those things generally considered sacred in some way. Red ochre found at ancient burial sites hints at the hope for a renewal of life. The colour red has become synonymous with the preservation of our life-force, as in the logos of the Red Cross and Red Crescent. Danger signs and signals are also often surrounded in red or coloured red to indicate warning of the loss of life. Fire has two facets. It can be a warming life-saver or an uncontrollable destroyer. In our daily lives, too much red energy will harm or exhaust us; too little and we have no energy for any activity. Too much red energy and we become over involved in the workings of the material world; too little and we find the world a threatening and dangerous place that we need to escape from.

Red at a physical level relates to the circulation of the blood through the body that provides our cells with oxygen (fuel) and nutrients (food). To provide red energy we need to exercise and eat in a way that maximises this to the full. If we eat too little or continuously exhaust ourselves physically and mentally, not only does this process break down, we also stress our adrenal glands. These glands control our ability to respond to survival situations by pumping hormones into our bloodstream, heightening senses and reaction times. If we overstretch our bodies for too long, this natural reaction becomes a permanent state, which eventually leads the whole system into a state of collapse. Classical "red" exercise involves using the lower limbs – walking, running, swimming or bicycling, which when carried out for about 20 minutes, increases the oxygen supply to our cells.

Massaging the legs or feet can do the same. Eating red coloured foods and foods rich in minerals can increase the amount of energy that is available to us.

Below: red, symbolised by fire, has two facets. It can be a warming life-saver or an uncontrollable destroyer.

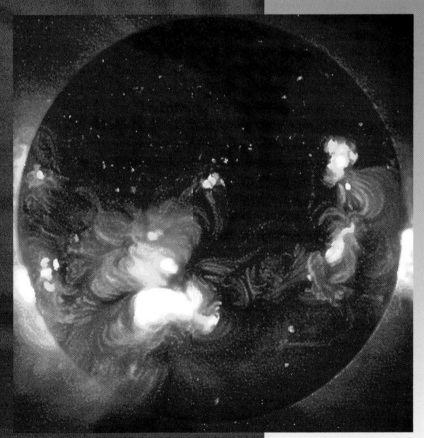

Any direct expression of emotion is linked to the colour red. Anger and passion especially have both traditionally been thought of as "red" emotions and phrases like "red light district" and "red-in-the-face" have crept into everyday speech to reinforce this. The characteristics of "red" emotions are their strength, their immediacy and their short duration. Many societies avoid or refuse to accept the expression of these emotions. This produces people who feel guilty about being angry or deny their passion. Wearing red clothing or carrying red crystals can help to overcome this or it can sometimes be easier to introduce something red into the living space. Flower essences such as scarlet pimpernel, hazel or oak can also be used to ease the expression of red feelings.

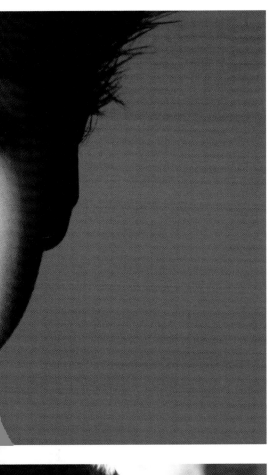

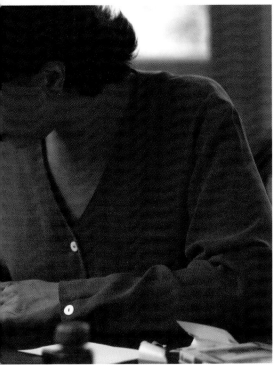

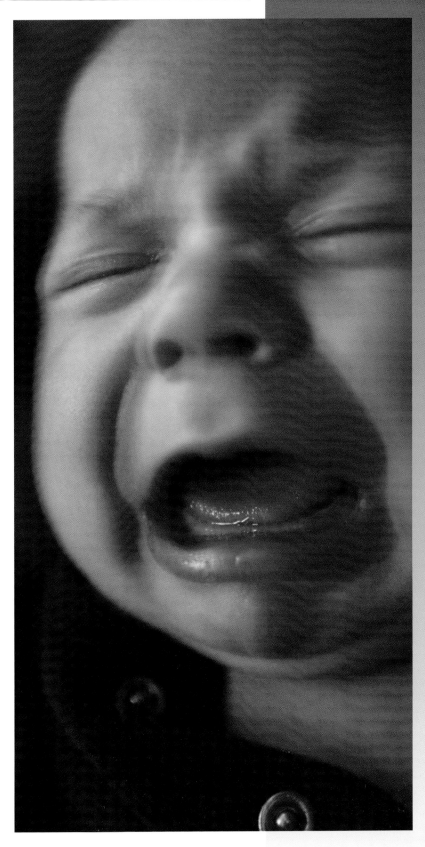

On a mental level, the drive to start new projects and to create foundations for new business is related to red. The energy that drives innovators and entrepreneurs is seldom adapted to the management of stable businesses, so the initiator will often move on once the new project is working. It is not uncommon to see combined with this level of initiative a very assertive character that needs to be impulsive, rash and daring. Here the person continuously challenges or tests themselves to reinforce their living and survival skills. When mental energy is low, visualising red or eating red energy foods can help, (coffee and tea both provide "red" energy), though too much increases irritability and can create addictive behaviour.

Right: coffee and tea both provide "red" energy, though too much increases irritability and can create addictive behaviour.

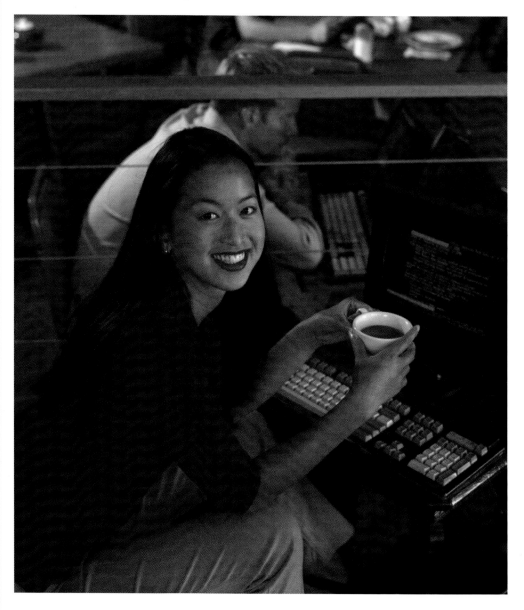

On a spiritual level, red reminds us that no matter how spiritually inclined we may be, we are dependent on the survival and well-being of our physical body as a tool with which to express that spirituality in the world. Wearing red, eating red foods or foods rich in minerals, exercising, releasing our strong feelings and occasionally acting on impulse all reaffirm our connection through our bodies to the material world.

SUMMARY:

To increase or balance the red energy in your life:

Wear red clothes.

Eat red-coloured foods or foods that supply red energy (remember - coffee, tea, sugar and chocolate are only temporary "fixes").

Use red crystals:
garnet, red jasper, ruby

Use essential oils that have red energy:
ylang ylang, frankincense, black pepper

Use flower essences of red flowers;
scarlet pimpernel, red rose, hazel

Activities:
running, speed and field sports

Left and below: When mental energy is low, visualising red or eating red energy foods can help,

BROWN

Brown is mainly associated with the colour of soil and resonates well with all aspects of the natural world. Like the Earth, brown represents a solid background to our lives. Brown is a mixture of the palette primary colours red, yellow and blue, creating a comfortable and familiar colour.

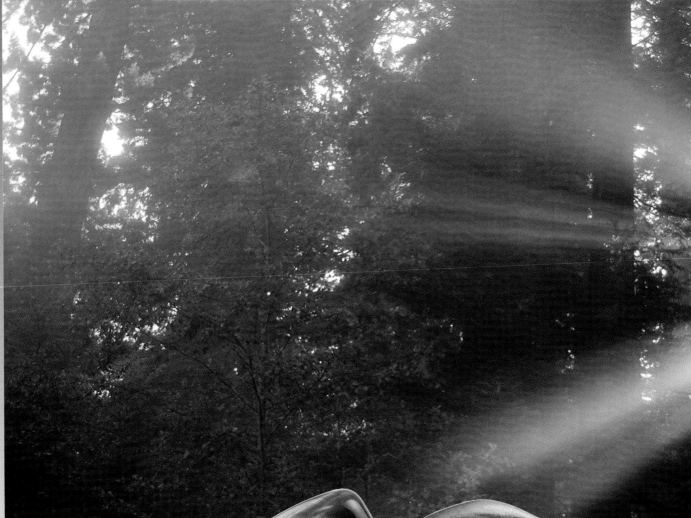

Above: brown is mainly associated with the colour of soil and resonates well with all aspects of the natural world.

Right: tiger's eye crystals.

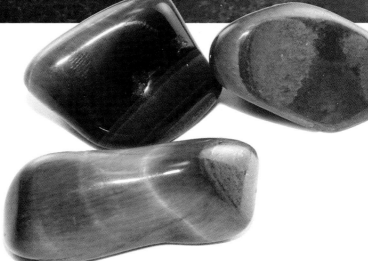

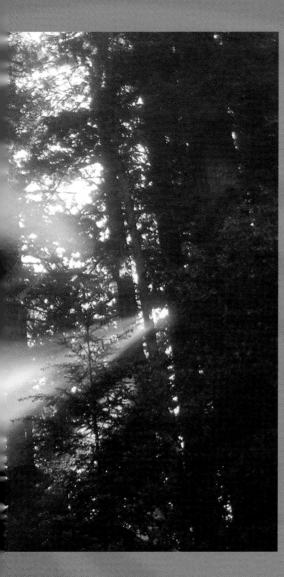

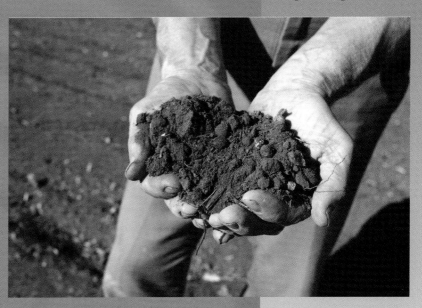

Below: introducing brown into physical activity occurs through nature-based actions, like gardening,

Through the association of the colour with the earth, brown suggests safety, free from the menace that black can suggest. Brown encourages the practical expression of skills that can take time to develop. The steady quality of brown ensures a thorough and accomplished outcome. Introducing brown into physical activity occurs through nature-based actions, like gardening, walking in woodland, crafting wood or working with clay. Wearing brown helps to maintain stability and reminds us of the need to be practical.

Right: brown is an excellent choice for surroundings involved with long-term study or logical thought processes. It helps ideas to become real, so very useful for the library or study of the visionary or inventor.

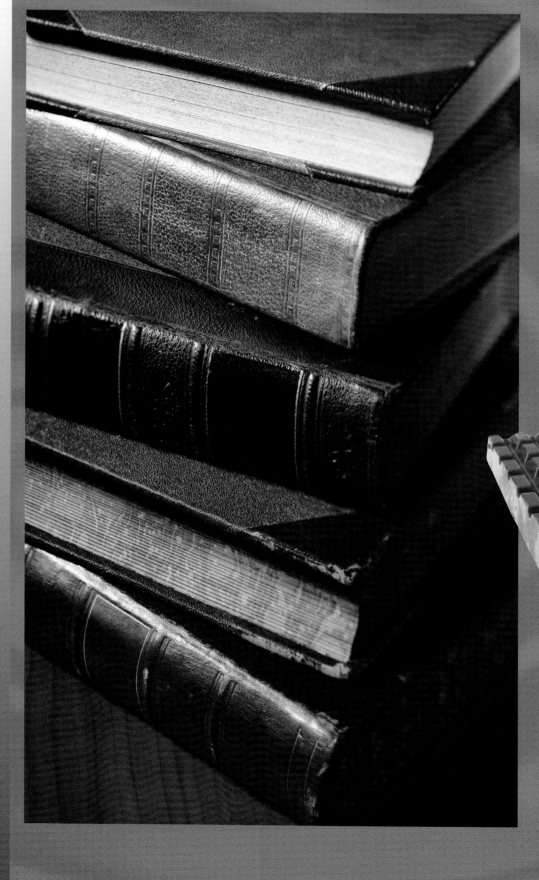

All tones and shades of brown calm the emotions. It can help us to feel more self-reliant. Like black, brown can also allow us to stay in the background and to remain detached from strong emotions. Other people often find brown non-threatening when it is used as a main dress colour, as it can help the wearer to look more approachable. Chocolate is well known as a food that creates a feeling of well-being for many. However, too much can become addictive. Other brown foods, like nuts, can provide the nutrients to stabilise the emotions without the short-lived buzz of sugar and cocoa.

Brown is an excellent choice for surroundings involved with long-term study or logical thought processes. It helps ideas to become real, so very useful for the library or study of the visionary or inventor. Without natural sunlight, brown can eventually dull the flow of original thought as it can create a strong need for stability and a love of routine. Brown can be used to help create new routines. Carrying brown crystals like tiger's eye or dark citrine can help here. Hazel nuts are rich in the nutrients that help the pathways in the brain to function well, ideal for periods of thought or study.

Below: chocolate is well known as a food that creates a feeling of well-being for many.

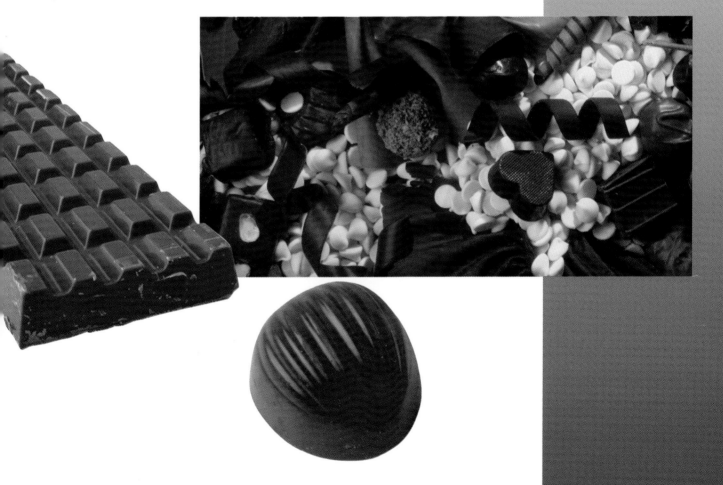

Below: bring some logical thought into your life by using wooden furntiure in certain areas of your home.

On a spiritual level, brown suggests an ability to integrate with one's surroundings. This encourages us to be content with where we are and who we are, free from unrealistic wishes. This type of integration takes time, patience and effort. Like the primary colour components that create brown, this integration will represent all facets of life and personality.

SUMMARY:

To increase or balance the brown energy in your life:

Wear brown clothes.

Use wood furniture in your home.

*Eat brown foods
(nuts, brown rice, seeds).*

Use brown crystals:

tiger's eye, dark citrine, staurolite, iron quartz

Activities:

walking, gardening, pottery, woodworking

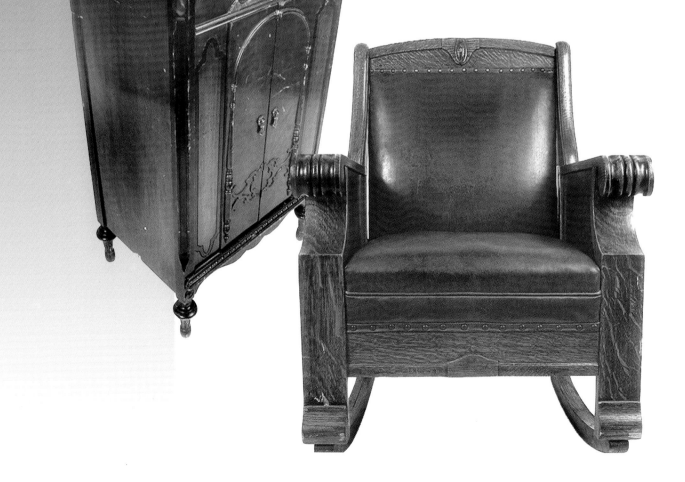

ORANGE

Orange is created from a blend of red and yellow in equal parts. The yellow content gives the powerful red energy the capacity to be directed and sustained. Orange has two qualities that function on all levels of our being. These are release and creativity, linked by the need for life-force to flow through us completely unhindered.

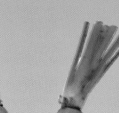

Below: orange foods can help detoxify the body and help the flow of energy.

In the physical body orange is related to the lower abdomen in general, but to the large intestine and reproductive organs in particular. The large intestine deals with the ability to release by the elimination of waste products, the reproductive organs are concerned with fertility. Without the ability to release waste products from the body efficiently, the system becomes constipated and toxic. Eating orange foods (apricots, oranges, carrots) and foods that relate to orange qualities (brown rice, foods high in natural roughage, oats), can reduce the incidence of such problems. Massaging the lower abdomen and back with oils that carry an orange vibration (neroli, sandalwood) can help to relieve symptoms. The ability to create something real from our dreams, ideas and inspiration works through the orange energy. The bodily function of reproduction is only one facet of this creativity. Children of the emotions, the mind and our dreams are also gestated and born here. Musicians, artists, and dancers all use a lot of orange energy. When creative energy gets blocked it can be released by using orange. Wearing orange, eating orange foods, massaging "orange" oils, orange items within the environment will all ease the flow of energy. Flower essences from orange-coloured or orange-smelling flowers, such as marigold and mock orange, can also play their part. When a system becomes static or blocked, not only is constipation present on all levels, but there is lack of creativity, too. If the physical symptoms in either area persist, the underlying emotional and mental problems linked to orange need to be addressed.

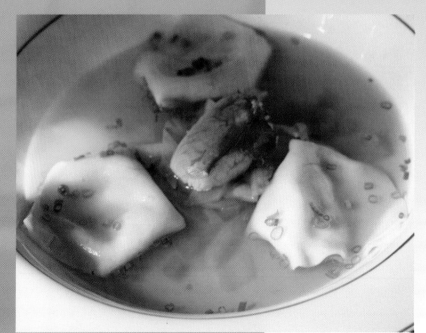

Right: orange releases the creativity of the artist.

Far right: musicians, artists, and dancers all use a lot of orange energy. When creative energy gets blocked it can be released by using orange.

Orange on the emotional level links the extremes of fun and pleasure with shock and trauma. When we shut off the enjoyment of life for any reason, orange in any form can be a difficult colour to settle with. Strict social mores concerning personal pleasure, desire and enjoyment, repress and inhibit the flow of orange energy through the body, creating blocks of guilt on all levels – physical, emotional, mental and spiritual. The same effect occurs after experiencing trauma, particularly if we felt powerless. In these cases, orange can be uncomfortable as it tends to remind us that something needs to be dealt with.

If orange can be introduced carefully, in any form, it can bring about the healing that is needed. When we are unwilling or unable to let go of memories or problems, we can experience a sort of emotional constipation and excessively tense muscles. This can lead to the physical problem of constipation, urinary difficulties and tenderness in the lower abdomen or back.

On the level of the mind orange releases the creativity of the artist. This is not just about formulating ideas, but bringing them to fruition in a way that enhances beauty and elicits appreciation from others. This can be achieved through any medium so long as it brings pleasure, release and relaxation.

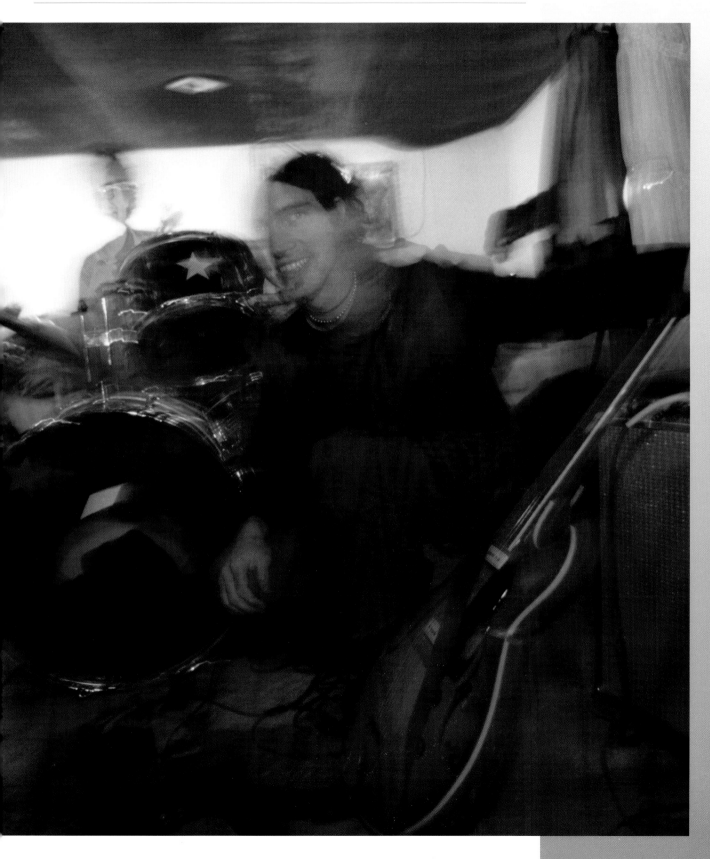

Below: using flower essences made from marigold or Californian poppy will all help orange energy.

On a spiritual level, orange represents the subtle blueprint of our physical bodies, often referred to as the etheric layer, or that part of the aura that is closest to the physical body. In this layer, the model for our physical body is held. If our physical, emotional or mental bodies become damaged, the etheric does too. Effective healing will repair the etheric. If the etheric is not repaired, pain can remain or the physical body never completely heals because the template or model is incomplete. Use of any sort of orange will keep the energy and information held in the etheric free of blocks, leaving the physical body to complete its healing and to release stress effectively.

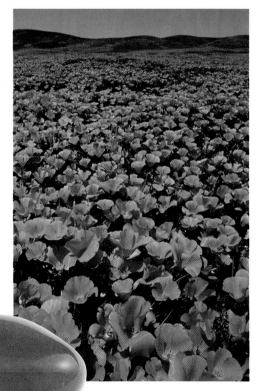

Below: carnelian crystals.

SUMMARY:

To increase or balance the orange energy in your life:

Wear some orange clothing.

Eat orange foods (oranges, apricots, peaches) or foods that create an orange effect (brown rice, oats, sesame seeds, vitamin C, zinc).

Use orange crystals:
carnelian, dark citrine or crystals that work in an orange way (dark opal, Herkimer diamond, selenite)

Use orange essential oils:
neroli, mandarin, cedar

Use flower essences made from orange flowers:
marigold, Californian poppy

Activities:
music, dancing, any form of art

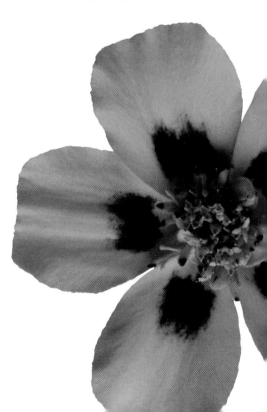

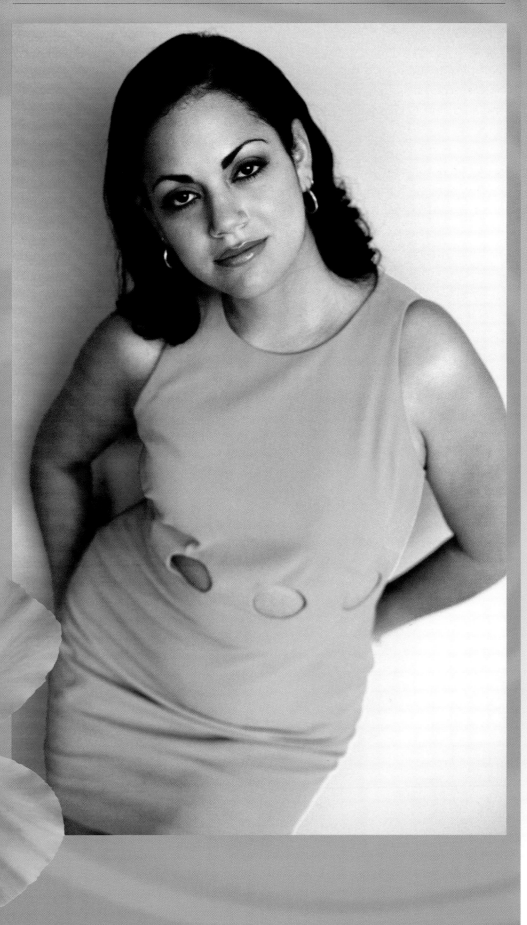

Left: wearing something orange will increase or balance the orange energy in your life.

68

GOLD

Below: the mineral gold has been sought after or fought over for centuries, because acquiring vast amounts is indicative of wealth and status.

When a mix of red and yellow favours the yellow, the rich tones of gold emerge. Our instinctive reactions to gold in our surroundings shows us, possibly more than any other colour, how universal human reactions to colour are. The mineral gold has been sought after or fought over (on the battle field and in the boardroom) because acquiring vast amounts is indicative of wealth and status. Gold is a commodity that powerful people would like to control as its rarity reflects those qualities of "worth" and "value" that are most highly regarded.

The colour gold when shone onto the body soothes nerves and encourages the body to relax, as does the visual impact of the colour. Minute amounts of the mineral gold are required for optimum functioning of the nervous system. Gold resonates with the skin, the largest organ of the body, and creams made from gold-coloured flowers, (chamomile, marigold, evening primrose) and gold-coloured natural oils (vitamin E) are used to heal minor damage to the skin and to help to keep the skin supple.

Left: creams made from gold-coloured flowers are used to heal minor damage to the skin and to help to keep the skin supple.

Below: taking time out to play and have fun is an important part of gold energy.

The link that gold has with our emotions highlight the qualities of contentment and comfort. Wearing gold brings a degree of self-awareness and confidence that gets people noticed. In a small amount gold can suggest wealth and good taste, whereas too much hints at a need to impress. This demarcation between a class act and a shyster showman is very subtle. Individuals through the ages have all fallen foul of what is acceptable show and what is judged to be pride and boastfulness. In a state of balance, gold can create and project a lazy emotional style that is a comfortable and secure place to be.

There is a natural leadership quality associated with gold at a mental level – to be a successful leader there has to be an ability to carry the weight of the inevitable attention, preferably without the ego becoming too large. If the balance of gold is lost, an egotistical, proud dictator emerges who, ironically, denies everyone else their gold qualities of happiness, relaxation and contentment. It is important not to get complacent with success but to somehow keep it fresh and untarnished. Taking time out to play and have fun is an important part of gold energy.

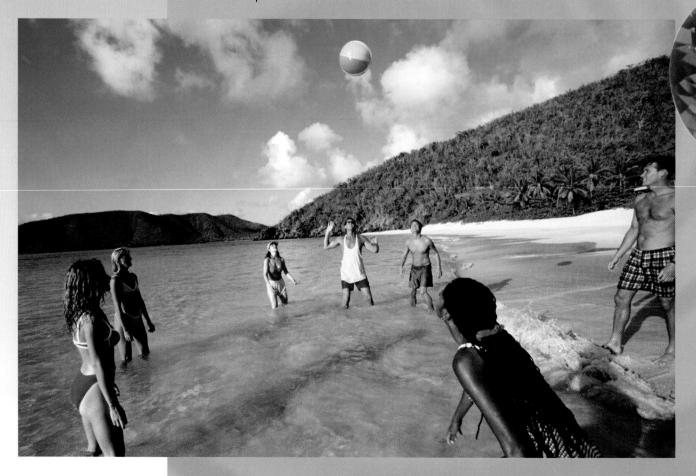

At a spiritual level, gold suggests a serene, wise and well-rounded personality. It is easy to assume that someone with gold energy at a spiritual level "has it made" and there is nothing else to be achieved. However, like a swan on a pond, the elegant vision of ease hides furious paddling. Gold at this level shows that constant vigilance and hard work directed at self-development and self-healing pays off – but never stops.

SUMMARY:

To increase or balance the gold energy in your life:

Have something of golden colour in your immediate environment.

Eat foods that bring warmth to the body – spicy foods, ginger.

Take time out to play in the sunshine.

Wear gold jewellery – amber, rich citrine, gold topaz.

Use herbs and nutrients like vitamin E, dandelion.

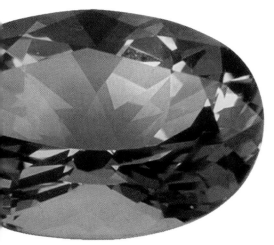

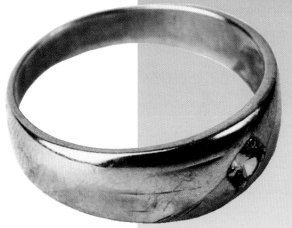

Below: to help the flow of gold energy wear gold jewellry.

Left: citrine.

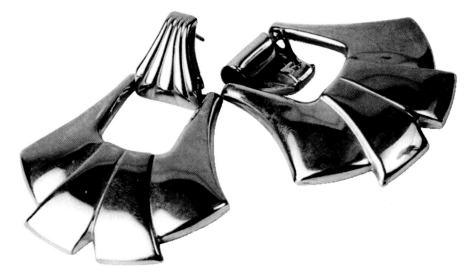

YELLOW

The bright, crisp yellows have an invigorating effect compared to the cosy shades of gold. Yellow is linked to the ability to make decisions from the given information. The richest source of yellow is the light from the bright sun (in the main part of the day). If we exclude natural light from our lives, for whatever reason, be it work or illness, we cut ourselves off from one of the greatest sources of healing.

Below: yellow has an invigorating effect compared to the cosy shades of gold.

In our physical bodies yellow relates to our digestive, nervous and immune systems. All of these systems depend on correct information being available and the subsequent correct choices being made. Our digestive system breaks down the food we eat into constituents that our bodies identify and absorb for our health and growth. If the digestive system's decisions go awry, we experience digestive problems and poor absorption of nutrients. The nervous system relays information to our brain where it is sifted, filed and acted upon when necessary. If the nervous system cannot prioritise, confusion and fear increase. The immune system identifies and destroys cells it considers harmful to the body. If the immune system mis-identifies cells, it fails to fight viruses, bacteria and other invading cells or identifies harmless items as something that needs to be fought as occurs with allergies or, in the other extreme, fights our own healthy body cells by mistake (auto-immune diseases). Many of us need extra yellow to combat the pressures of living in the 21st century. Wearing yellow may not always be popular, but yellow in our homes, yellow foods, food supplements and herbs that resonate with yellow (vitamin B, evening primrose oil, vitamin E, St. John's wort) can all help.

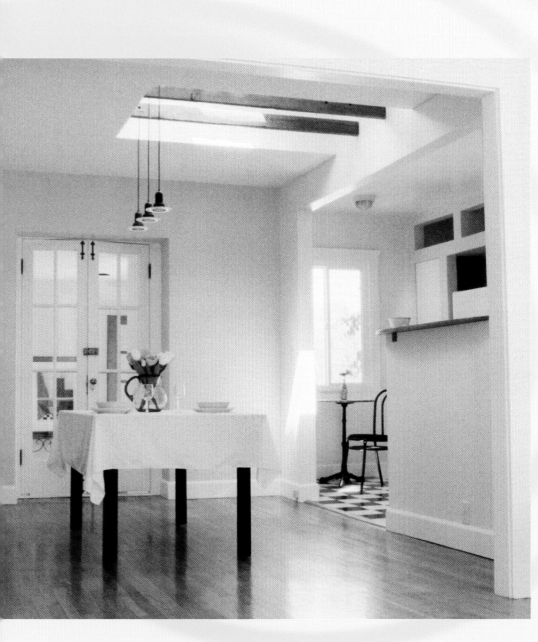

Left: the richest source of yellow is the light from the bright sun, but we can introduce yellow into our homes in many ways to help balance or increase yellow energy.

Many people who find themselves mentally and emotionally stressed can be so as a result of problems created by the physical imbalances of yellow. Unfortunately we live in an age where information dominates our society and the processes of logic and science are considered vital. We work in artificial light often surrounded by electrical machines. All of this depletes yellow energy. As the body becomes more stressed, thinking patterns start to fail. Without yellow it is difficult to concentrate, study or remember things we know that we know. Enhancing yellow helps the ability to discriminate and judge what is needed. Without a balance of yellow at an emotional and mental level, we strive for an unreachable perfection instead of accepting our best efforts.

Spiritually, yellow represents the ability to know who and what we are. With this ability we can deflect the unwanted attention of others and unwanted energy from machines in our environment. If we cannot differentiate between ourselves and our surroundings, we become dominated by things outside of ourselves, and we feel powerless and weak.

Above: eat yellow food such as bananas to help combat the pressures of living in the 21st century.

Right: lemon quartz.

SUMMARY:
To increase or balance the yellow energy in your life:

Wear yellow.

Introduce yellow into your surroundings.

Eat yellow foods (bananas, grains, citrus fruits), and foods rich in vitamins.

Supplement your diet with vitamin B complex, vitamin E, or the herb St. John's wort, evening primrose oil.

Sunbathe for short periods.

Use crystals;
lemon quartz, yellow citrine, yellow fluorite

Use flower essences from yellow flowers:
daffodil, crocus, marigold, chrysanthemum, hypericum

Our eyes are especially sensitive to all shade and tints of green. Green is in the middle of the visible spectrum and epitomises the qualities of balance and harmony. It is the colour we relate to nature, trees and plants and to a way of life that works in harmony with the Earth.

In nature, we see the physical expression of green in the new shoots of plant growth in the spring. This is part of the natural cycle of birth and death that we readily accept in nature but can have problems accepting in our lives. The processes of life and growth inevitably involve the death of one cycle, so that another can emerge. This creates the balance. For any growth and development to be sustainable, each stage builds on what has gone before. When we have problems working with or accepting this, a walk in a park, a forest or by the sea can bring back our perspective. Whether vegetarian, vegan or carnivore, we all depend in some way on the plant kingdom for our food. Reverence for all life helps to keep our perspective in harmony with reality. In our physical bodies, green relates to the heart, lungs, the arms and hands. The heart and lungs are organs that rhythmically expand and contract, in a cycle of renewal and elimination that we depend on to live. The arms and hands, we use to pull things and people towards us, for closer inspection, to hold or relate to. We also use them to push things away from us when we feel we no longer want or need them in our lives.

Left: we see the physical expression of green in the new shoots of plant growth in the spring.

Emotionally green is a way of relating to everyone and everything in the environment. It is necessary to balance personal requirements with the needs of others. In personal relationships this dynamic is an ever-changing set of polarities. We seem to explore the extremes before settling on the balance – weighing freedom against inhibition and repression, caring and love against manipulation, control and dominance against encouragement. Emotions constantly change and we can be misled if we expect emotions to be the same all the time. Like the heart and lungs, the process of letting go and holding in never stops. Security cannot be achieved emotionally, as emotions fluctuate as part of their natural function. Knowing ourselves, life-experience and practice can help us to deal with this natural cycle. When we feel overwhelmed emotionally the opportunity to be in natural surroundings is not always possible. Using essential oils like rosemary, lavender or pine in an oil-burner can help to create green energy and a new sense of personal space.

Mentally, green suggests the patterns and cycles of our thought processes. When we are young, we take our guidance and behaviour models from those who set the rules. This is fine as it helps us to become secure in our homes and immediate surroundings. As we mature, we reach a point where we need to take on the process of setting our boundaries and patterns of behaviour ourselves, accepting the new responsibility that comes along with it. Breaking away from the patterns and ties of childhood is not easy, but unless this happens we are unable to grow into independent adults. It is usually better for this "breaking away" to happen when there is a chance to take a break from the normal flow of our lives, as this gives time to explore the new possibilities. At these times wearing green can be very supportive. Many people instinctively bring more green into their lives at these times – even eating only green foods for a few days can encourage changes in our thinking.

Above: green jade stones; wear jade jewellry (right), to balance or increase the green energy in your life.

Far right: green is the colour we relate to nature, trees and plants and to a way of life that works in harmony with the Earth. Emotionally green is a way of relating to everyone and everything in the environment.

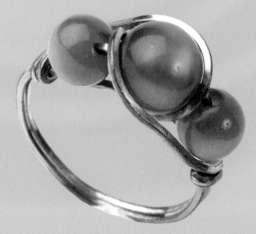

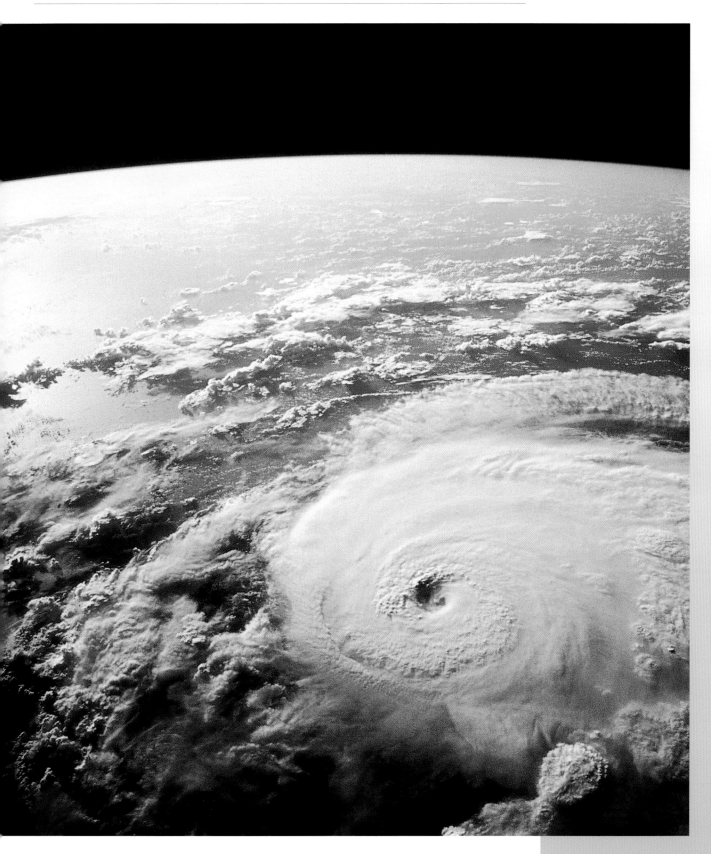

Below: wearing green and eating green foods such as apples will improve your green energy.

Below right: walking in the countryside and being near trees will enhance your green energy

On a spiritual level, green suggests the capacity to "do your own thing" regardless of what everyone else says or does. This confirms that at this level we are unique rather than deliberately eccentric or rebellious. No-one can live our lives for us. We can take advice, but ultimately we are responsible for ourselves. Accepting this can free an individual, which in turn gives the opportunity for others to release themselves from any duty of care they might feel they had for that person. Everyone can then move on to the next phase of growth.

SUMMARY:

To increase or balance the green energy in your life:

Wear green clothes.

Eat green foods (leafy vegetables, apples, pears etc.).

Walk in the countryside, around trees or sit in the garden.

Use crystals:
e.g. aventurine, emerald, green jasper, jade, tourmaline

Use flower essences made from tree flowers:
e.g. lime, maple, willow

Use any essential oils

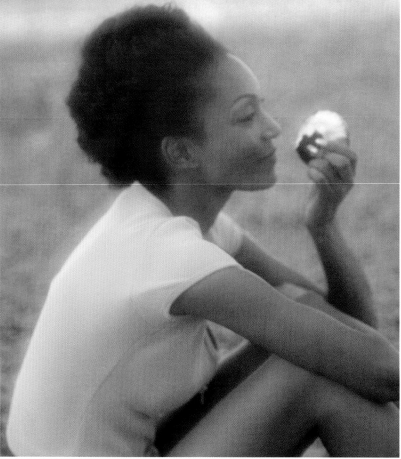

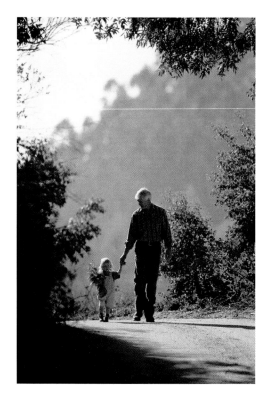

TURQUOISE

Turquoise is a beautiful blend of blue and green. It was named after the Turks who decorated their buildings in tiles of this colour. When this colour appears in nature, most people find it very attractive and calming. Turquoise creates an easy flow of energy through the physical body that helps relaxation, not just physically, but also emotionally. Working particularly on the upper chest, turquoise can help to deepen breathing and relax tense muscles in and around the shoulders and upper back. This in turn helps the thymus gland to function correctly, aiding our immune system to withstand the pressures of living in the present day.

On an emotional level, turquoise helps the true expression of personal emotions. This reflects the true individuality of the person. For many, this aspect of turquoise is difficult to accept. Wearing turquoise-coloured clothes or bringing the colour into the home as furnishings or wall colour can help if self-expression is a difficult thing. The resurgence and popularity of this colour in the 1990s reflected the growth in diverse spiritual philosophies.

Below: turquoise creates an easy flow of energy through the physical body that helps relaxation.

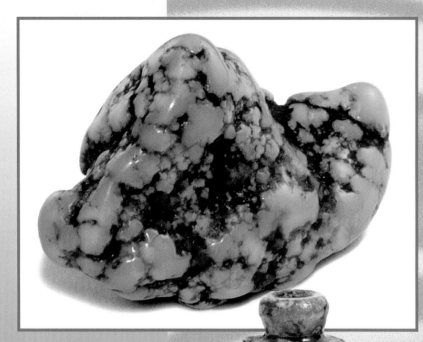

Mentally, turquoise epitomises the opportunity to express or interpret old ideas in new and relevant ways. It can be a useful colour to wear when needing to take a stand over an issue that is felt strongly about or when it seems difficult to fit easily into the surroundings.

On a spiritual level, turquoise is very protective. The mineral turquoise has been greatly valued in the parts of the world where it occurs naturally. Historically it has been used for both protection and healing, for instance turquoise amulets or jewellery.

SUMMARY:

To increase or balance turquoise in your life:

Wear some turquoise-coloured clothes.

Wear turquoise jewellery or carry a piece in your pocket.

Try to say what you feel and not what you think people want to hear.

Above and right: turquoise, is very protective and is greatly valued in the parts of the world where it occurs naturally.

Far right: wear some turquoise coloured clothing when you need to make a stand over an issue you feel strongly about.

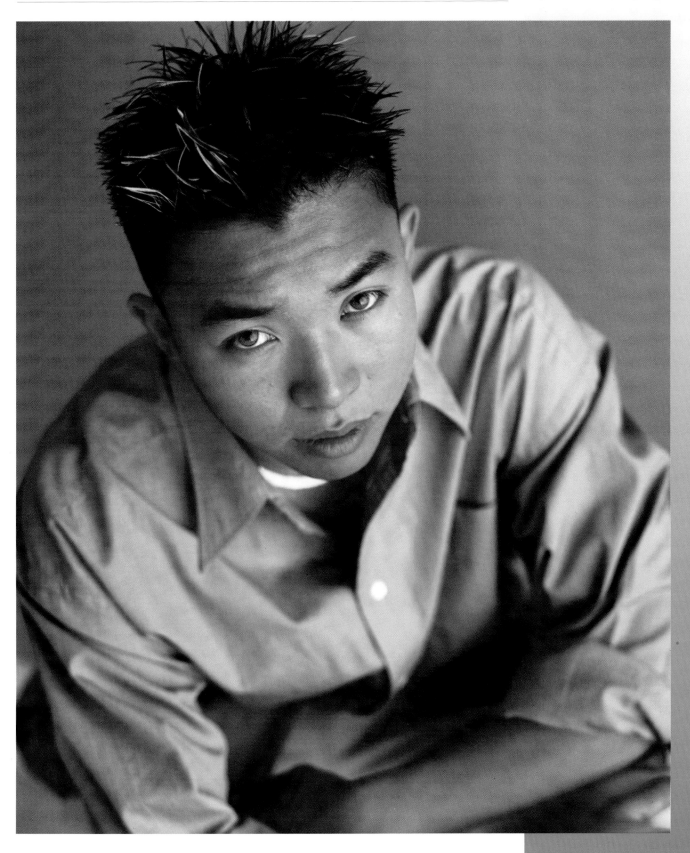

BLUE

Below: the dark blue on a clear starry nigh instills wonder as does the bright blue on a clear sunny day.

Gazing up at the sky on a sunny day or at the stars on a clear night, the blues, one bright and one very dark, can both instil wonder, peace and an appreciation of the vastness of space and the universe. Across all bands of experience, blue indicates a flow of energy. This can be communication, love or information. The direction of that flow is always from a state of high intensity or pressure towards one that is lower. For example, someone with knowledge of a subject will teach or instruct someone with less knowledge. The process can be described as a flow of information from one person to the other, and this is related to the colour blue.

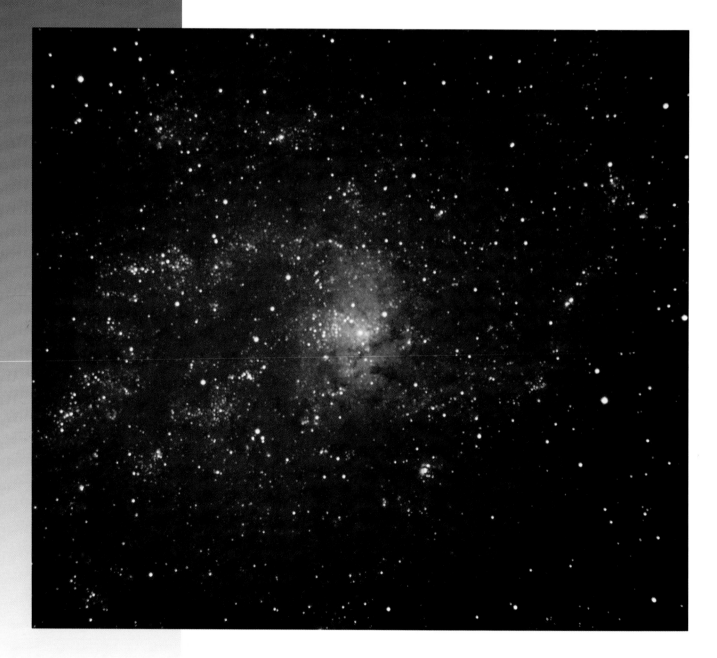

Blue has a sedating effect on the physical body. Shining blue light onto the body has been used to reduce inflammation and swelling in joints and other tissues. It will calm any situation down when used for short periods. If used in lighting for too long, though, it can become depressive and cold. Blue is also linked closely to communication of all sorts. The most common sort is verbal communication – language, speech, singing and laughter – but it also includes non-verbal skills and body language. When communication of any sort is prevented or inhibited, the natural flow stops. This creates a build-up of pressure that we often experience as frustration or disappointment. Since blue is related to the ears, eyes, nose and throat, inhibiting the flow of energy can create physical problems in these areas. If you are prevented from speaking out, sore throats, earache and a stiff neck could be the physical result. If this should occur, wearing a blue scarf or tie around the neck or carrying blue crystals can reduce some of the more uncomfortable symptoms. Arnica, the classical homoeopathy remedy for trauma, acts as a "blue energy", as it brings flow into a situation that has become stuck through shock.

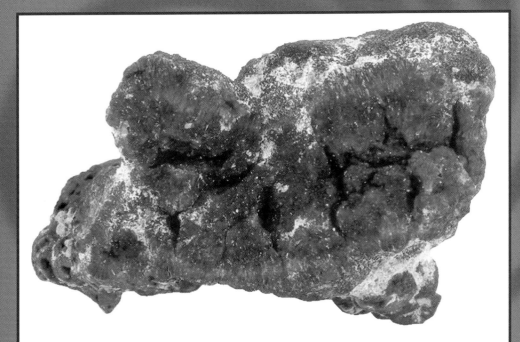

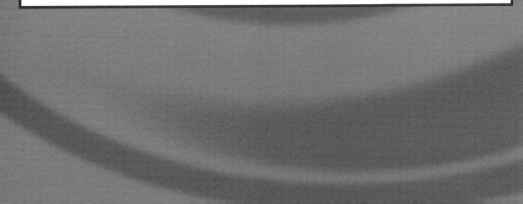

Left: if you are prevented from speaking out, sore throats, earache and a stiff neck could be the physical result, carrying a blue crystal such as azurite can reduce these symptoms.

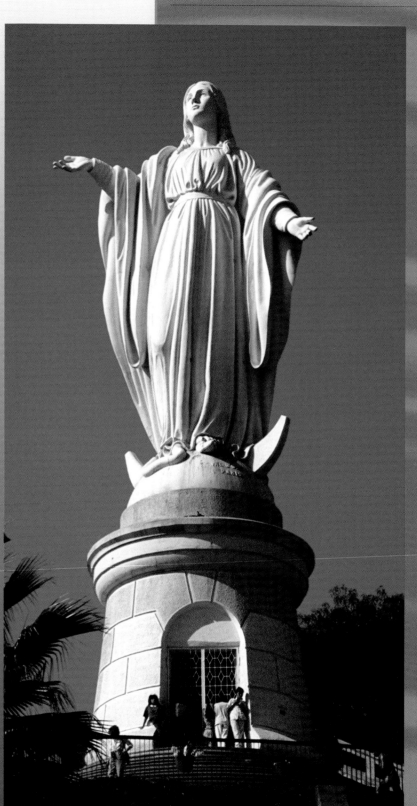

For thousands of years blue has been associated with objects or people of devotion (the Virgin Mary and Krishna). Here devotion is directed towards a powerful emotional source. This flow of devotion can bring the attributes of these beings closer to the lives of people. Blue can also calm our emotions, allowing thoughts to separate from ordinary levels of communication. Many old places of worship have blue stained-glass windows or blue décor to help this process along. The homoepathic remedy aconite come from a plant with intense blue flowers and is an excellent remedy for acutely painful situations of all sorts.

The flow of mental energy and communication related to blue moves to provide a clarity of knowledge and understanding. Both teaching and learning, especially associated with philosophy, religion and further education, are linked to blue. Blue therefore becomes an ideal colour to wear if you want to instil confidence in others and to be thought of as someone who is reliable and trustworthy. Sometimes the speed of information is such that we can have sudden ideas or intuitions that, if followed, will change our lives. These seem to come from outside of our normal mental functions, and are sometimes thought of as coming from an infinite or divine source.

Blue represents the realm of subtle perception at a spiritual level. These skills include clairvoyance (clear seeing), clairaudience (clear hearing), and clairsentience (clear feeling). Skills such as mediumship and the ability to channel information from other sources also relate to the darker shades of blue. All of these can be seen purely as an information flow from one source to another, but from a more unworldly source than day-to-day communication and conversation. For these types of skills to become secure and stable, the energies of the complementary colour orange and the grounding energy of red are both needed.

SUMMARY:

If you want to balance or increase the blue energy in your life:

Take time to look up at a starry night sky or a clear blue sky on a sunny day.

Wear blue clothes and introduce small amounts of blue into your environment,

Use essential oils like:

rosemary, lavender, blue chamomile

Use flower essences from blue flowers:

bluebell, harebell, forget-me-not, scabious

Use crystals:

celestite, blue topaz, sapphire, lapis lazuli, sodalite, azurite

Far left: for thousands of years blue has been associated with objects or people of devotion such as the Virgin Mary.

Below: to increase or balance blue energy, use blue crystals such as lapis lazuli (left), sodalite (right) and saphire (centre).

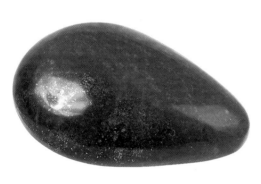

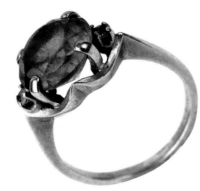

VIOLET

Hundreds of years ago, violet and purple dyes were very expensive commodities and were reserved for use by the ruling classes, the clergy and the rich. Today shades and tints of violet are often thought of as the "most spiritual" colours, mostly based on their historical use. For well-being, though, we need all colours and no one colour is more important or spiritual than any other. The tradition that links violet with healing is explained by its blend of red and blue, the opposite ends of the visible spectrum. A body will take from violet light the energy it needs, so violet can be applied in any situation to help to create well-being.

Right: emotions that resonate with violet – sympathy, empathy and the ability to see other people's points of view – are revealed by those who work in selfless service for others.

Below: use amethyst crystals to help synchronise your body.

Violet is related to the head. Its constituent colours of red and blue represent the different and opposite functions of the left and right hemispheres of the brain. The left hemisphere is linked to logical thought and outward expression, the right hemisphere to creativity and absorption of information. The degree of balance between the hemispheres is seen in an individual's ability to co-ordinate physical movement and other activities that need the left and right sides of the body to work in synchronistic harmony. Amethyst, a violet type of quartz, is thought to help this process, as is diamond and fluorite. Amethyst, placed on the head, may help at the onset of migraine headaches, and can reduce their severity.

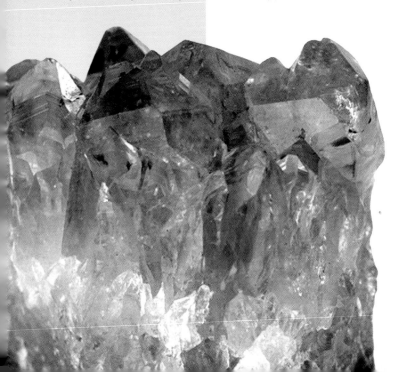

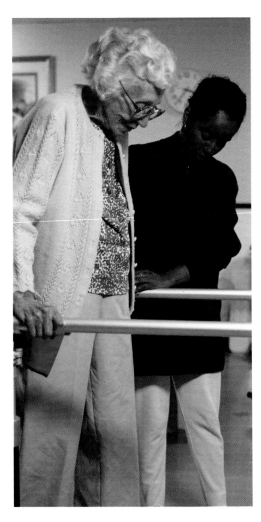

Emotions that resonate with violet – sympathy, empathy and the ability to see other people's points of view – are revealed by those who work in selfless service for others. Violet, however, can also show the opposite facet of its energy very easily. This becomes apparent where people martyr themselves for others, not from a healthy and altruistic stance, but from a lack of self-worth. Helpers can see others as more needy or deserving and so sacrifice themselves. Viewed from a broad perspective, this is a type of negative-egotism. A more balanced standpoint is to help others to the maximum of one's ability as well as looking after your own well-being. This way the service can be carried on indefinitely as it derives from a stable emotional base. The complementary colour to violet, yellow, and its quality of self-knowledge, helps to stop the violet energy from becoming unworldly. Violet is the colour of imagination and inspiration. However, all too easily, these positive traits can distort and become fantasy and delusion. Holding the positive balance requires input from all the other colours of the spectrum and their accompanying skills. The sleight of hand of the magician can amaze, yet the same energy in a trickster can disgust.

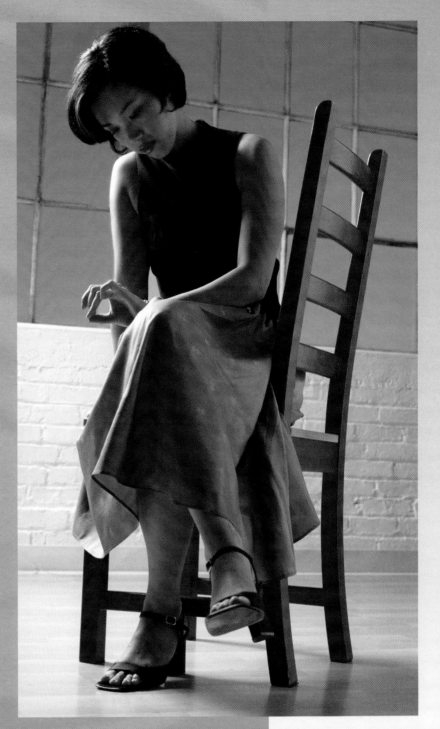

Above: to increase or balance the violet energy in your life wear violet clothes.

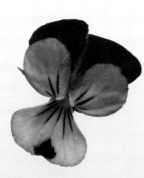

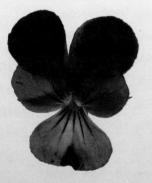

Above: use flower essences of pansies or violets to increase the violet energy.

Below: amethyst.

Violet as a spiritual energy relates to the integration of the spiritual aspects of life with the mundane and practical. Many teachers and gurus say that it is pointless having high ideals and views if we cannot apply them in our daily lives. This is the challenge of violet. Bringing these two aspects together can be achieved most easily through some sort of ritual. Whatever you choose to do – regular attendance to a place of worship, daily personal prayers or giving thanks for a beautiful day – if it is done from the heart with sincerity, it is very powerful. Incense, special clothes and specific foods can all create a sacred atmosphere to connect and integrate with your inner being.

SUMMARY:

To increase or balance the violet energy in your life:

Wear violet clothes.

Use crystals:
amethyst, sugilite, violet fluorite, diamond, charoite

Use essential oils:
lavender, violet

Use flower essences of violet flowers:
violet, pansy, petunia, lavender, gentian etc.

Examine your motives for getting involved in healing, charities and groups.

PINK

Pink is usually just a combination of red and white, but some deeper shades also have a hint of blue. The amount of red present in each mix will indicate the amount of life-force or practical energy present. Red relates to the motivation to drive ourselves to accomplish and white suggests that all things are possible. Pink can be thought of as supporting whatever the individual does in relationship to everything and everyone else.

Wearing pink is often thought of as a feminine prerogative, yet in many Eastern cultures, red represents the female energy and white, the male energy. We have a tendency to regard pink as a very gentle ineffective colour which could not be further from reality. Whereas violet balances the spectrum extremes of red and blue, pink harmonises the gender polarities of male and female, or Yang and Yin, expressive and receptive. Keeping a piece of rose quartz as a room decoration can help to balance the energies of the environment, though it would be need to be cleansed regularly. Deeper shades of pink, especially the rich "bubble-gum" colour, are able to stabilise subtle personal energies, whether it is worn as clothing, jewellery or is introduced into room décor.

Deep magenta has also been found to calm aggressive behaviour when people are exposed to the colour for short periods (10 minutes). Longer exposure seems, however, to emphasise more of the "red" component and to increase agitation. The paler pinks link more closely to attitudes we hold about

ourselves, e.g. self-worth, self-tolerance and self-esteem. Many people are able to express love for others more easily than they can for themselves. Forgiving others often comes more easily if we have come to forgive ourselves first. A high level of self-acceptance comes from facing the fears we have about ourselves.

Below: forgiving others often comes more easily if we have come to forgive ourselves first; pink energy helps with this.

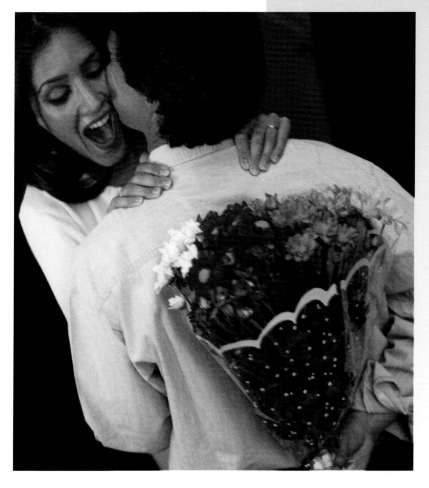

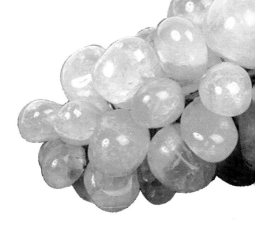

Above: rose quartz.

Far right: To increase or balance the pink energy in your life wear a shade of pink you feel comfortable with.

Rose quartz as a healing crystal is often thought to be very gentle, but the impact of Pink healing may not be easy to deal with without an emotional release.

All the "self" issues come from beliefs that we hold about ourselves and the world. When we see ourselves as separate or polarised from the world, we tend to hold negative attitudes about ourselves. A very common attitude is the undervaluing of personal skills and roles in society. Visualising pink around ourselves can ease difficult situations. When we feel threatened by particular people, imagining pink around them can also help to take fear out of the interaction.

For many people pink is the colour of "unconditional love". This type of love is difficult for most humans to express if they are really honest with themselves. Compassion, however, allows for our human frailties and foibles. Compassion is not weak. The red/white mix of pink suggests the strength needed to be really compassionate. It takes a strong person to stand back and allow someone to learn to be who they are. Compassion isn't rushing in and trying to "fix" everything or make it "right". Compassion is accepting what "is", with all the responsibility, pain and joy it can bring.

SUMMARY:

To increase or balance the pink energy in your life:

Wear a shade of pink you feel comfortable with.

Use pink crystals:
Rose quartz, rhodonite, rhodocrosite

Use essential oils:
rose, rose geranium

Use flower essences of pink flowers:
flowering currant, geranium, red campion etc.

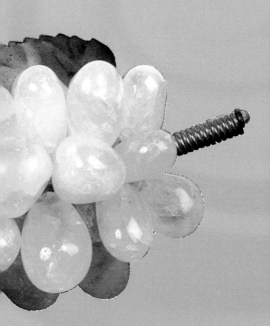

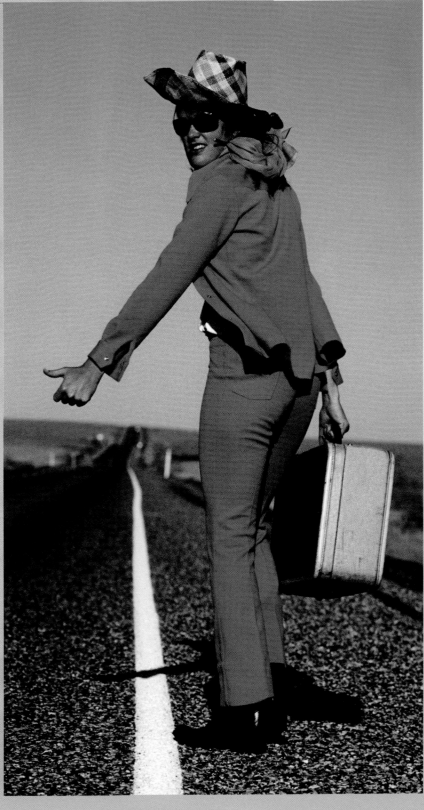

WHITE

White is not necessarily thought of as a colour. White occurs when the whole spectrum of light is seen together or when red, yellow and blue light is mixed. Everything is present in white, nothing is hidden or secret. White is thought to have a very cold quality, as in snow, or an extremely hot quality, such as burning metal. Either can be life-threatening and can remind us of death and the ending of things. White can also denote purity, holiness and cleanliness. White is a colour that sets things apart from the rainbow spectrum of everyday life. In ceremonies white can add a special quality, so beginnings and endings of lives or life changes are often symbolised by white – the end of one cycle and the beginning of another.

Below: the stark reality of white in the physical world hints at its uncompromising nature.

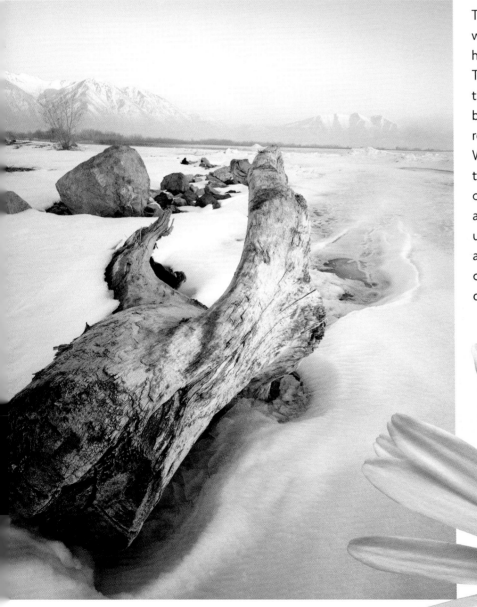

The stark reality of white in the physical world (for example, snow, old bones) hints at its uncompromising nature. There is an openness and truth in white that some people find uncomfortable. It becomes a mirror-like experience, reflecting emotions back to their source. Wearing white can be a deliberate device to set yourself apart from or above others, making any approach difficult and therefore possibly creating unnecessary fear or suspicion. The addition of a small amount of another colour to white will make a huge difference to the response from others.

The core energy of white is direct and impersonal. It can represent rapid transformation and complete change. Its ability to purify what it connects with is unsurpassed. Without another colour to soften it, though, white can be an uncomfortable experience. Flower essences made from white flowers (Star of Bethlehem, stitchwort, daisy, snowdrop) can help to create profound changes in emotional and mental patterns. Clear and white crystals tend to work in the same way and are excellent transmuters and transmitters of energy.

SUMMARY:

To increase or balance the white energy in your life:

Wear white with another colour of your choice.

Fast for a day, drinking only water.

Use clear and white crystals:

e.g. clear quartz, moonstone, opal, diamond

Use flower essences of white flowers:

Star of Bethlehem, cherry laurel, daisy, snowdrop, apple, nettle

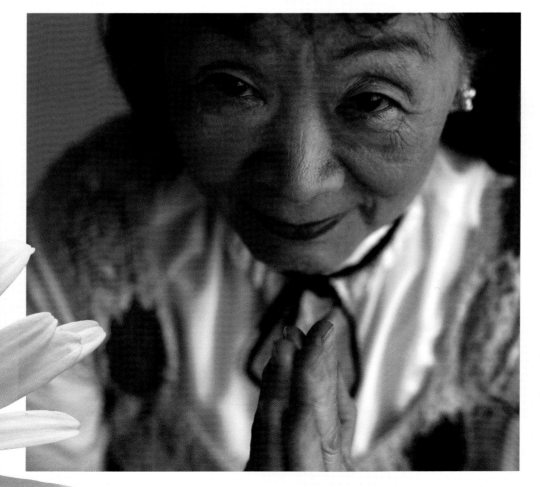

Left: when wearing white the addition of a small amount of another colour will make a huge difference to the response from others.

far left: flower essences made from white flowers such as daisy, can help to create changes in emotional and mental patterns.

INDEX

INDEX

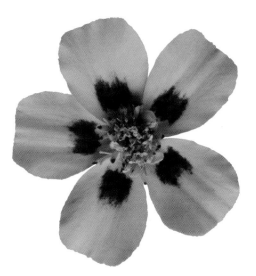